HEALTH CARE ISSUES, COSTS AND ACCESS

MILITARY HEALTH CARE

HEALTH CARE ISSUES, COSTS AND ACCESS

Additional books in this series can be found on Nova's website under the Series tab.

Additional E-books in this series can be found on Nova's website under the E-book tab.

MILITARY AND VETERAN ISSUES

Additional books in this series can be found on Nova's website under the Series tab.

Additional E-books in this series can be found on Nova's website under the E-book tab.

HEALTH CARE ISSUES, COSTS AND ACCESS

MILITARY HEALTH CARE

BRIAN M. GAGLIARDI
EDITOR

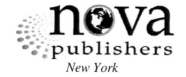

publishers
New York

Library of Congress Cataloging-in-Publication Data

ISBN: 978-1-62417-339-4

Published by Nova Science Publishers, Inc. ✝ New York

CONTENTS

PREFACE

The primary objective of the military health system, which includes the Defense Department's hospitals, clinics, and medical personnel, is to maintain the health of military personnel so they can carry out their military missions and to be prepared to deliver health care during wartime. The military health system also covers dependents of active duty personnel, military retirees and their dependents, including members of the reserve components. This book provides an overview of how the military health system is structured; a description of TRICARE and who is eligible; the costs of military health care to beneficiaries; the relationship of TRICARE to Medicare; and whether the Affordable Care Act (ACA) affects TRICARE.

Chapter 1 - The primary objective of the military health system, which includes the Defense Department's hospitals, clinics, and medical personnel, is to maintain the health of military personnel so they can carry out their military missions and to be prepared to deliver health care during wartime. The military health system also covers dependents of active duty personnel, military retirees and their dependents, including some members of the reserve components. The military health system provides health care services through either Department of Defense (DOD) medical facilities, known as "military treatment facilities" or "MTFs" as space is available, or through private health care providers. The military health system currently includes some 56 hospitals and 365 clinics serving 9.7 million beneficiaries. It operates worldwide and employs some 58,369 civilians and 86,007 military personnel.

Since 1966, civilian care to millions of dependents and retirees (and retirees' dependents) has been provided through a program still known in law as the Civilian Health and Medical Program of the Uniformed Services (CHAMPUS), but more commonly known as TRICARE. TRICARE has four main benefit plans: a health maintenance organization option (TRICARE Prime), a preferred provider option (TRICARE Extra), a fee-for-service option (TRICARE Standard), and a Medicare wrap-around option (TRICARE for Life) for Medicare-eligible retirees. Other TRICARE plans include TRICARE Young Adult, TRICARE Reserve Select and TRICARE Retired Reserve. TRICARE also includes a pharmacy program and optional dental plans. Options available to beneficiaries vary by the beneficiary's duty status and location.

Chapter 2 - The 111th Congress passed, and the President signed into law, the Patient Protection and Affordable Care Act (P.L. 111-148; ACA), as amended by the Health Care and Education Reconciliation Act of 2010 (P.L. 111-152; HCERA), and hereafter referred to as ACA. In general, ACA did not make any significant changes to the Department of Defense (DOD) TRICARE program or to the Department of Veterans Affairs (VA) health care system. However, many have sought clarification as to whether certain provisions in ACA, such as a mandate for most individuals to have health insurance, or extending dependant coverage up to age 26, would apply to TRICARE and VA health care beneficiaries.

To address some of these concerns, Congress has introduced and/or enacted legislation. The TRICARE Affirmation Act (H.R. 4887; P.L. 111-159), signed into law on April 26, 2010, affirms that TRICARE satisfies the minimum acceptable coverage requirement in ACA. Similarly, P.L. 111-173, signed into law on May 27, 2010, clarifies that the Civilian Health and Medical Program of the Department of Veterans Affairs (CHAMPVA), Spina Bifida Health Care Program, and the Children of Women Vietnam Veterans Health Care Program meet the "minimum essential coverage" requirement under ACA. TRICARE coverage of children was extended to age 26 by the Ike Skelton National Defense Authorization Act for Fiscal Year 2011 (P.L. 111-383).

Chapter 3 - TRICARE Reserve Select (TRS) provides certain members of the Selected Reserve—reservists considered essential to wartime missions—with the ability to purchase health care coverage under the Department of Defense's (DOD) TRICARE program after their active duty coverage expires. TRS is similar to TRICARE Standard, a fee-forservice option, and TRICARE Extra, a preferred provider option.

The National Defense Authorization Act for Fiscal Year 2008 directed GAO to review TRS education and access to care for TRS beneficiaries. This report examines (1) how DOD ensures that members of the Selected Reserve are informed about TRS and (2) how DOD monitors and evaluates access to civilian providers for TRS beneficiaries. GAO reviewed and analyzed documents and evaluated an analysis of claims conducted by DOD. GAO also interviewed officials with the TRICARE Management Activity (TMA), the DOD entity responsible for managing TRICARE; the regional TRICARE contractors; the Office of Reserve Affairs; and the seven reserve components.

Chapter 4 - The Department of Defense (DOD) provides health care through its TRICARE program, which is managed by the TRICARE Management Activity (TMA). TRICARE offers three basic options. Beneficiaries who choose TRICARE Prime, an option that uses civilian provider networks, must enroll. TRICARE beneficiaries who do not enroll in this option may obtain care from nonnetwork providers under TRICARE Standard or from network providers under TRICARE Extra.

The National Defense Authorization Act for Fiscal Year 2008 directed GAO to evaluate various aspects of beneficiaries' access to care under the TRICARE Standard and Extra options. This report examines (1) impediments to TRICARE Standard and Extra beneficiaries' access to civilian health care and mental health care providers and TMA's actions to address the impediments; (2) TMA's efforts to monitor access to civilian providers for TRICARE Standard and Extra beneficiaries; (3) how TMA informs network and nonnetwork civilian providers about TRICARE Standard and Extra; and (4) how TMA informs TRICARE Standard and Extra beneficiaries about their options. To address these objectives, GAO reviewed and analyzed TMA and TRICARE contractor data and documents. GAO also interviewed TMA officials, including those in its regional offices, as well as its contractors.

Chapter 5 - In 1993, President Clinton modified the military policy on providing abortions at military medical facilities. Under the change directed by the President, military medical facilities were allowed to perform abortions if paid for entirely with non-Department of Defense (DOD) funds (i.e., privately funded). Although arguably consistent with statutory language barring the use of Defense Department funds, the President's policy overturned a former interpretation of existing law barring the availability of these services. On December 1, 1995, H.R. 2126, the FY1996 DOD appropriations act, became law (P.L. 104-61). Included in this law was language barring the use of funds to administer any policy that permits the performance of abortions at any DOD facility except where the life of the mother would be endangered if the fetus were carried to term or where the pregnancy resulted from an act of rape or incest. Language was also included in the FY1996 DOD Authorization Act (P.L. 104-106, February 10, 1996) prohibiting the use of DOD facilities in the performance of abortions. These served to reverse the President's 1993 policy change. Recent attempts to change or modify these laws have failed.

Over the last three decades, the availability of abortion services at military medical facilities has been subjected to numerous changes and interpretations. Within the last 15 years, Congress has considered numerous amendments to effectuate such changes. Although Congress, in 1992, passed one such amendment to make abortions available at overseas installations, it was vetoed.

In: Military Health Care
Editor: Brian M. Gagliardi

ISBN: 978-1-62417-339-4
© 2013 Nova Science Publishers, Inc.

Chapter 1

MILITARY MEDICAL CARE: QUESTIONS AND ANSWERS[*]

Don J. Jansen and Katherine Blakeley

SUMMARY

The primary objective of the military health system, which includes the Defense Department's hospitals, clinics, and medical personnel, is to maintain the health of military personnel so they can carry out their military missions and to be prepared to deliver health care during wartime. The military health system also covers dependents of active duty personnel, military retirees and their dependents, including some members of the reserve components. The military health system provides health care services through either Department of Defense (DOD) medical facilities, known as "military treatment facilities" or "MTFs" as space is available, or through private health care providers. The military health system currently includes some 56 hospitals and 365 clinics serving 9.7 million beneficiaries. It operates worldwide and employs some 58,369 civilians and 86,007 military personnel.

Since 1966, civilian care to millions of dependents and retirees (and retirees' dependents) has been provided through a program still known in law as the Civilian Health and Medical Program of the Uniformed Services

---

[*] This is an edited, reformatted and augmented version of the Congressional Research Service Publication, CRS Report for Congress RL33537, dated September 27, 2012.

(CHAMPUS), but more commonly known as TRICARE. TRICARE has four main benefit plans: a health maintenance organization option (TRICARE Prime), a preferred provider option (TRICARE Extra), a fee-for-service option (TRICARE Standard), and a Medicare wrap-around option (TRICARE for Life) for Medicare-eligible retirees. Other TRICARE plans include TRICARE Young Adult, TRICARE Reserve Select and TRICARE Retired Reserve. TRICARE also includes a pharmacy program and optional dental plans. Options available to beneficiaries vary by the beneficiary's duty status and location.

This report answers several frequently asked questions about military health care, including:

- How is the military health system structured?
- What is TRICARE?
- What are the different TRICARE plans and who is eligible?
- What are the costs of military health care to beneficiaries?
- What is the relationship of TRICARE to Medicare?
- How does the Affordable Care Act affect TRICARE?
- What are the long-term trends in defense health care costs?
- What is the Medicare Eligible Retiree Health Care fund, which funds TRICARE for Life?

The Government Accountability Office (GAO) and the Congressional Budget Office (CBO) have also published important studies on the organization, coordination and costs of the military health system, as well as its effectiveness addressing particular health challenges. The Office of the Assistant Secretary of Defense for Health Affairs Home Page, available at http://www.health.mil/, may also be of interest for additional information on the military health system.

BACKGROUND

Since 1966, civilian care to millions of dependents and retirees (and retirees' dependents) has been provided through a program still known in law as the Civilian Health and Medical Program of the Uniformed Services (CHAMPUS), but more commonly known as TRICARE. TRICARE has four main benefit plans: a health maintenance organization option (TRICARE

Prime), a preferred provider option (TRICARE Extra), a fee-for-service option (TRICARE Standard), and a Medicare wrap-around option (TRICARE for Life) for Medicare-eligible retirees. Other TRICARE plans include TRICARE Young Adult, TRICARE Reserve Select and TRICARE Retired Reserve. TRICARE also includes a pharmacy program and optional dental plans. Options available to beneficiaries vary by the beneficiary's duty status and location.

The Government Accountability Office (GAO) and the Congressional Budget Office (CBO) have also published important studies on the organization, coordination and costs of the military health system, as well as its effectiveness addressing particular health challenges. The Office of the Assistant Secretary of Defense for Health Affairs Home Page, available at http://www.health.mil/, may also be of interest for additional information on the military health system.

QUESTIONS AND ANSWERS

1. How Is the Military Health System Structured?

Administrative Structure

The military health system consists of (1) the Defense Health Program (DHP) which is centrally directed by the Office of the Secretary of Defense and executed by the military departments, and (2) medical resources under the direction of the combatant or support command within the military departments. For DOD, the Assistant Secretary of Defense for Health Affairs (ASD(HA)) controls non-deployable medical resources, facilities and personnel. The ASD(HA) reports to the Under Secretary of Defense for Personnel and Readiness who reports to the Deputy Secretary of Defense. The following all currently report to the ASD/HA:

- Deputy Assistant Secretary of Defense for Clinical and Program Policy
- Deputy Assistant Secretary of Defense for Force Health Protection and Readiness
- Deputy Assistant Secretary of Defense for Health Budget and Financial Policy
- Deputy Director TRICARE Management Activity

- Chief Information Officer for Health
- Director, Strategy and Development
- Director, Communication and Media Relations
- Director, Defense Center of Excellence for Psychological Health and Traumatic Brain Injury
- President, Uniformed Services University of the Health Sciences

Other elements within the Office of the Secretary of Defense, such as the Office of the Director for Program Analysis and Evaluation and the Office of the Under Secretary of Defense (Comptroller), are also responsible for various aspects of the military health system.

Within the services, the Surgeons General of the Army, Navy and Air Force retain considerable responsibility for managing military medical facilities and personnel. The Joint Staff Surgeon advises the Chairman of the Joint Chiefs of Staff.

The Surgeon General of the Army heads the U.S. Army Medical Command (MEDCOM) which along with the Office of the Surgeon General itself compose the Army Medical Department (AMEDD). The Surgeon General of the Army reports directly to the Secretary of the Army. MEDCOM commands fixed hospitals and other AMEDD commands and agencies. Field medical units, however, are under the command of the combat commanders.

The Surgeon General of the Navy reports to the Chief of Naval Operations through the Chief, Navy Staff and Vice Chief of Naval Operations and heads the Navy Bureau of Medicine and Surgery (BUMED), the headquarters command for Navy Medicine. All Defense Health Program resources allocated to the DON are administered by BUMED. Also within the Department of the Navy, the Medical Officer, U.S. Marine Corps advises the Commandant of the Marine Corps and Headquarters staff agencies on all matters about health services.

The Surgeon General of the Air Force serves as functional manager of the U.S. Air Force Medical Service, an element of Headquarters, U.S. Air Force. The Air Force Surgeon General advises the Secretary of the Air Force and Air Force Chief of Staff.

Potential Consolidation

The Final Report of the Task Force on Future of Military Health Care noted in 2007 that there has been considerable debate about the appropriate command and control structure for the military health system.[1] The current organizational structure has been observed by some to present an opportunity to gain efficiencies and save costs by consolidating administrative, management, and clinical functions. Alternatives to the current structure that have been suggested include a defense health agency or a unified medical command. Section 716 of the National Defense Authorization Act for Fiscal Year 2012 (P.L. 112-81) required the Secretary of Defense to submit to the congressional defense committees a report on military health system reorganization options. DOD's report, submitted March 2, 2012, considered 12 options and recommended Defense Health Agency with Service Military Treatment Facilities (MTFs) (similar to the current system) reporting that all of the Unified Medical Command options would increase costs.

Medical Personnel and Facilities

The military health system currently includes 56 hospitals and 365 clinics serving 9.7 million beneficiaries. It operates worldwide and employs some 58,369 civilians and 86,007 military personnel. Direct care costs include the provision of medical care directly to beneficiaries, the administrative requirements of a large medical establishment, and maintaining a capability to provide medical care to combat forces in case of hostilities. Civilian providers under contract to DOD have constituted a major portion of the defense health effort in recent years.

TRICARE Organization

The TRICARE Management Activity (TMA) listed above supervises and administers the TRICARE program. TMA is organized into six geographic health service regions:

- TRICARE North Region covering Connecticut, Delaware, the District of Columbia, Illinois, Indiana, Kentucky, Maine, Maryland, Massachusetts, Michigan, New Hampshire, New Jersey, New York, North Carolina, Ohio, Pennsylvania, Rhode Island, Vermont, Virginia, West Virginia, Wisconsin, and portions of Iowa, Missouri, and Tennessee. The TRICARE North regional contractor is currently Health Net Federal Services.
- TRICARE South Region covering Alabama, Arkansas, Florida, Georgia, Louisiana, Mississippi, Oklahoma, South Carolina, and most of Tennessee and Texas. The TRICARE South regional contractor is currently Humana Military Health Services.
- TRICARE West Region covering Alaska, Arizona, California, Colorado, Hawaii, Idaho, most of Iowa, Kansas, Minnesota, most of

Missouri, Montana, Nebraska, Nevada, New Mexico, North Dakota, Oregon, South Dakota, portions of Texas, Utah, Washington, and Wyoming. The TRICARE West regional contractor is TriWest Healthcare Alliance.

- TRICARE Europe Area covering Europe, Africa, and the Middle East.
- TRICARE Latin America and Canada Area covering Central and South America, the Caribbean Basin, Canada, Puerto Rico and the Virgin Islands.
- TRICARE Pacific Area covering Guam, Japan, Korea, Asia, New Zealand, India and Western Pacific remote countries.

More information is available at http://www.TRICARE.mil/tma/About TMA.aspx.

2. What Is the Unified Medical Budget?

ASD(HA) prepares and submits a unified medical budget which includes resources for the medical activities under his or her control within the DOD. The unified medical budget includes funding for all fixed medical treatment facilities/activities, including such costs as real property maintenance, environmental compliance, minor construction and base operations support. Funds for medical personnel and accrual payments to the Medicare Eligible Retiree Health Care Fund (MERHCF - see "3. What is the Medicare Eligible Retiree Health Care Fund (MERHCF)?," below) are also included. The unified medical budget does not include resources associated with combat support medical units/activities. In these instances the funding responsibility is assigned to military service combatant or support commands.

Unified medical budget funding has traditionally been appropriated in several places:

- The defense appropriations bill provides Operation and Maintenance (O&M), Procurement, and Research, Development, Test and Evaluation (RDT&E) funding under the heading "Defense Health Program."
- Funding for military medical personnel (doctors, corpsmen, and other health care providers) and TRICARE for Life accrual payments are

generally provided in the defense appropriations bill under the "Military Personnel" (MILPERS) title.

- Funding for medical military construction (MILCON) is generally provided under the "Department of Defense" title of the military construction and veterans affairs bill.
- A standing authorization for transfers from the MERHCF to reimburse TRICARE for the cost of services provided to Medicare eligible retirees is provided by 10 U.S.C. 1113.
- Costs of war-related military health care are generally funded through supplemental appropriations bills.

Other resources are made available to the military health system from third-party collections authorized by 10 U.S.C. 1097b(b) and a number of other reimbursable program and transfer authorities. The President's budget typically refers to the unified medical budget request as its funding request for the military health system but only includes an exhibit for the DHP in the "Department of Defense - Military" chapter and exhibits for the MERHCF in the "Other Defense—Civil Programs" chapter of the Appendix volume. Medical MILCON and MILPERS request levels are generally found in DOD's budget submissions to Congress.

As illustrated in **Figure 1** below, the Obama Administration's FY2013 unified medical budget request[2] totals $48.7 billion and includes:

- $32.5 billion for the Defense Health Program (not including "Wounded, Ill, and Injured" funding);
- $8.5 billion for military personnel;
- $1.0 billion for medical military construction; and
- $6.7 billion for accrual payments to the MERHCF.

Much more detailed breakouts are available in budget exhibits published by the Department of Defense at http://www.budget.mil.

3. What Is the Medicare Eligible Retiree Health Care Fund (MERHCF)?

The Floyd D. Spence National Defense Authorization Act for Fiscal Year 2001(P.L. 106-398) directed the establishment of the Medicare-Eligible Retiree Health Care Fund to pay for Medicare-eligible retiree health care beginning on October 1, 2002, via a new program called TRICARE for Life. Prior to this date, care for Medicare-eligible beneficiaries was space-available care in MTFs. The MERHCF covers Medicare-eligible beneficiaries, regardless of age.

The FY2001 NDAA also established an independent three-member DOD Medicare-Eligible Retiree Health Care Board of Actuaries appointed by the Secretary of Defense. Accrual deposits into the Fund are made by the agencies who employ future beneficiaries (DOD and the other uniformed services including the Public Health Service, the Coast Guard, and the National Oceanic & Atmospheric Administration) based upon estimates of future TRICARE for Life expenses. Transfers out are made to the Defense Health Program based on estimates of the cost of care actually provided each year. As of September 30, 2011, the Fund had assets of over $163.6 billion to cover future expenses.[3]

The Board is required to review the actuarial status of the fund; to report annually to the Secretary of Defense, and to report to the President and Congress on the status of the fund at least every four years. The DOD Office of the Actuary provides all technical and administrative support to the Board. Within DOD, the Office of the Under Secretary of Defense for Personnel and Readiness, through the Office of the Assistant Secretary of Defense (OASD) for Health Affairs (HA) has as one of its missions operational oversight of the defense health program including management of the MERHCF. The Defense Finance and Accounting Service provides accounting and investment services for the fund.

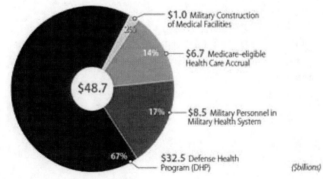

Source: Department of Defense FY2013 Budget Request Overview. Adapted by CRS Graphics.

Figure 1. FY 2013 Unified Medical Budget Request ($billions).

4. What Is TRICARE?

The Dependents Medical Care Act of 1956[4] provided a statutory basis for dependents of active duty members, retirees, and dependents of retirees to seek care at MTFs. Prior to this time, authority for such care was fragmented. The 1956 Act allowed DOD to contract for a health insurance plan for coverage of civilian hospital services for active duty dependents. Due to growing use of MTFs by eligible civilians and resource constraints, Congress adopted the Military Medical Benefits Amendments in 1966[5], which allowed DOD to contract with civilian health providers to provide non-hospital-based care to eligible dependents and retirees. Since 1966, civilian care to millions of dependents and retirees (and retirees' dependents) has been provided through a program still known in law as the Civilian Health and Medical Program of the Uniformed Services (CHAMPUS), but since 1994 more commonly known as TRICARE.

TRICARE has four main benefit plans: a health maintenance organization option (TRICARE Prime), a preferred provider option (TRICARE Extra), a fee-for-service option (TRICARE Standard), and a Medicare wrap-around option (TRICARE for Life) for Medicare-eligible retirees. Other TRICARE plans include TRICARE Young Adult, TRICARE Reserve Select and TRICARE Retired Reserve. These plans are described below. TRICARE also includes a Pharmacy program and optional dental plans. Options available to beneficiaries vary by the beneficiary's relationship to a sponsor, sponsor's duty status, and location.

5. What Are the Different TRICARE Plans?

TRICARE Prime
TRICARE Prime is a managed care option similar to a health maintenance organization—like such civilian arrangements, the plan's features include a primary care manager (either a military or a civilian health care provider) who oversees care and provides referrals to specialists. Referrals generally are required for such visits. To participate, beneficiaries must enroll and pay an annual enrollment fee, which is similar to an annual premium. Eligible beneficiaries may choose to enroll at any time. Enrollees receive first priority for appointments at military health care facilities and pay less out of pocket than do beneficiaries who use the other TRICARE plans. TRICARE Prime does not have an annual deductible.

Active duty service members are required to use TRICARE Prime. They and their family members, as well as surviving spouses (during the first three years), and surviving dependent children are exempt from the annual enrollment fee. Retired service members, their families, surviving spouses (after the first three years), eligible former spouses, and others are required to pay an annual enrollment fee, which is applied to the annual catastrophic out-of-pocket-limit .TRICARE Prime annual enrollment fees for military retirees were increased in fiscal year 2012 for new enrollees for the first time since the program began. Moving forward, under 10 U.S.C. 1097(e) TRICARE Prime enrollment fees will be subject to increases each fiscal year based on the annual retirement pay cost-of-living adjustment for the calendar year. For fiscal year 2013 (October 1, 2012–September 30, 2013) this enrollment fee is $269.28 for an individual and $538.56 for individual plus family coverage.

TRICARE Standard

TRICARE Standard is a traditional fee-for-service (FFS) option that does not require beneficiaries to enroll in order to participate. TRICARE Standard plan allows participants to use authorized out-of-network civilian providers, but it also requires users to pay higher out-of-pocket costs, generally 25% of the allowable charge for retirees and 20% for active duty family members. TRICARE Standard requires an annual deductible of $150/individual or $300/family for family members of sponsors at E-5 & above and $50/$100 for E-4 & below. Beneficiaries who use the Standard option must pay any difference between a provider's billed charges and the rate of reimbursement allowed under the plan.

TRICARE Extra

TRICARE Extra is also available to TRICARE Standard beneficiaries. It also has no formal enrollment requirement and mirrors a civilian preferred provider network. Network providers agree to accept a reduced payment from TRICARE and to file all claims for participants. By using network providers under TRICARE Extra, beneficiaries reduce their copayments, in general, to 20% of the allowable charge for retirees and 15% for active duty family members.

TRICARE Reserve Select

The TRICARE Reserve Select program was authorized by Section 701 of the Ronald W. Reagan National Defense Authorization Act for Fiscal Year 2005 (P.L. 108-375) which enacted Section 1076d of Title 10, United States

Code. TRICARE Reserve Select is a premium-based health plan available worldwide for qualified Selected Reserve members of the Ready Reserve and their families. Service members are not eligible for TRICARE Reserve Select if they are on active duty orders, covered under the Transitional Assistance Management Program, or eligible for or enrolled in the Federal Employees Health Benefits Program (FEHBP) or currently covered under the FEHBP through a family member. TRICARE Reserve Select provides benefits similar to TRICARE Standard. The government subsidizes the cost of the program with members paying 28% of the cost of the program in the form of premiums. For calendar year 2012, TRICARE Reserve Select premiums are $54.35 per month for member only coverage, and $192.89 per month for member and family coverage. For calendar year 2013, premiums are $51.62 per month for member only coverage, and $195.81 per month for member and family coverage.

TRICARE Retired Reserve

Section 705 of the National Defense Authorization Act for Fiscal Year 2010 (P.L. 111-84) added a new Section 1076e to Title 10, United States Code to authorize a TRICARE coverage option for so-called "gray area" reservists, those who have retired but are too young to draw retirement pay. The program established under this authority is known as TRICARE Retired Reserve. Previously, such individuals were not eligible for any TRICARE coverage. This is a premium-based health plan that qualified retired members of the National Guard and Reserve under the age of 60 may purchase for themselves and eligible family members. It is similar to TRICARE Reserve Select, but differs in that there is no government subsidy as there is with TRICARE Reserve Select. As such, retired Reserve Component members who elect to purchase TRICARE Retired Reserve must pay the full cost of the calculated premium plus an additional administrative fee. Retired Reserve Component personnel who elect to participate in TRICARE Retired Reserve become eligible for the same TRICARE Standard, TRICARE Extra or TRICARE Prime options as active component retirees when the service member reaches age 60. Calendar year 2012 premiums for member only coverage are $419.72 per month and member-and-family premiums are $1,024.43 per month. Calendar year 2013 premiums for member only coverage are $402.11 per month and member-and-family premiums are $969.10 per month.

TRICARE Young Adult

Section 702 of the Ike Skelton National Defense Authorization Act for Fiscal Year 2011 (P.L. 111-383) amended Title 10, United States Code, to add a new Section 1110b, allowing unmarried children up to age 26, who are not otherwise eligible to enroll in an employer-sponsored plan, to purchase TRICARE coverage. The option established under this authority is known as "The TRICARE Young Adult Program."

Unlike insurance coverage mandated by the Patient Protection and Affordable Care Act (P.L. 111-148) the TRICARE Young Adult Program provides individual coverage, rather than coverage under a family plan. A separate premium is charged.

The law requires payment of a premium equal to the cost of the coverage as determined by the Secretary of Defense on an appropriate actuarial basis. For calendar year 2012 the monthly premium for a TRICARE Young Adult (TYA) Prime enrollment is $201 and $176 for a TYA Standard enrollment.

TRICARE for Life

TRICARE for Life was created as "wrap-around" coverage to Medicare-eligible military retirees by Section 712 of the Floyd D. Spence National Defense Authorization Act for Fiscal Year 2001 (P.L. 106-398). TRICARE for Life functions as a second payer to Medicare, paying out-of-pocket costs for medical services covered under Medicare for beneficiaries who are entitled to Medicare Part A based on age, disability, or end-stage renal disease (ESRD). The beneficiaries are also eligible for medical benefits covered by TRICARE but not by Medicare.

Prior to creation of the TRICARE for Life program, coverage for Medicare-eligible individuals was limited to space available care in military treatment facilities. In recognition of the requirement to enroll in Medicare Part B, TRICARE for Life cost-sharing with beneficiaries is limited and there is no enrollment charge.

In order to participate in TRICARE for Life, these TRICARE-eligible beneficiaries must enroll in and pay monthly premiums for Medicare Part B. TRICARE-eligible beneficiaries who are entitled to Medicare Part A based on age, disability, or ESRD, but decline Part B, lose eligibility for TRICARE benefits.[6] In addition, individuals who choose not to enroll in Medicare Part B upon becoming eligible may elect to do so later during an annual enrollment period; however, the Medicare Part B late enrollment penalty would apply.

6. How Much Does Military Health Care Cost Beneficiaries?

Active duty service members receive medical care at no cost. Other beneficiaries pay differing amounts depending on their status, the TRICARE option enrolled in, and where they receive care. The tables below illustrate the costs to beneficiaries.

Table 1. Selected TRICARE Fees for Active Duty Personnel, Eligible Reservists, and Dependents

	Prime	Extra & Standard	
Annual Deductible	None	$150/individual or $300/family for E-5 and above; $50/ individual or $100/family below E-5	
Annual Enrollment Fee	None	None	
Annual Out-of-Pocket Limit	$1,000/family per fiscal year	$1,000/family per fiscal year	
Fees for Medical Services		**in-network (TRICARE Extra)**	**out of network (TRICARE Standard)**
Civilian Outpatient Visit	None	15% of negotiated rate	20% of allowable charge
Emergency Room Visit	None	15% of negotiated rate	20% of allowable charge
Hospitalization	None	Greater of $25 per admission or $17.05/day.	Greater of $25 per admission or $17.05/day.
Civilian Inpatient Behavioral Health	None	Greater of $25 or $20/day.	Greater of $25 or $20/day.

Source: TRICARE web site. Beneficiary costs current as of October 1, 2012.

For out-of-pocket limits, please see http://www.tricare.mil/mybenefit/home/Costs/ HealthPlanCosts

For full beneficiary cost tables for TRICARE Standard and Extra, please see: http://www.tricare.mil/mybenefit/home/Costs/HealthPlanCosts/TRICAREStandar dExtra?

Table 2. Selected TRICARE Fees for Retirees under Age 65 and Their Dependents Prime Extra & Standard

	Prime	Extra & Standard	
Annual Deductible	None	$150/individual or $300/family	
Annual Enrollment Fee	$269.28/individual or $538.56/family	None	
Annual Out-of-Pocket Limit	$3,000/family per fiscal year	$3,000/family per fiscal year	
Fees for Medical Services		**in-network (TRICARE Extra)**	**out of network (TRICARE Standard)**
Civilian Outpatient Visit	$12/visit	20% of negotiated rate	25% of allowable charge
Emergency Room Visit	$30/visit	20% of negotiated rate	25% of allowable charge
Hospitalization	Greater of $11/day or $25	Lesser of $250/day or 25% of billed charges for institutional services, plus 20% of separately billed services	Lesser of $708/day or 25% of billed charges for institutional services, plus 25% of separately billed services
Civilian Inpatient Behavioral Health	$40/day, no charge for separately billed professional services	20% of total charge plus 20% of allowable charge for separately billed professional services	High-Volume Hospital: 25% of hospital-specific per diem Low-Volume Hospital: Lesser of $208 per day or 25% of billed charges

Source: TRICARE web site. Beneficiary costs current as of October 1, 2012.

For out-of-pocket limits, please see http://www.tricare.mil/mybenefit/home/Costs/ HealthPlanCosts

For full beneficiary cost tables for TRICARE Prime for non-active duty families, please see: http://www.tricare.mil/mybenefit/home/Costs/HealthPlanCosts/ TRICAREPrimeOptions/EnrollmentFees? and http://www.tricare.mil/mybenefit/ home/Costs/HealthPlanCosts/TRICAREPrimeOptions/NetworkCopayments?

For full beneficiary cost tables for TRICARE Standard and Extra, please see: http://www.tricare.mil/mybenefit/home/Costs/HealthPlanCosts/TRICAREStandar dExtra?

Table 3. Selected TRICARE Fees for Reserve Select and TRICARE Retired Reserve

	Reserve Select		Retired Reserve	
Annual Deductible	$150/individual or $300/family for E-5 and above; $50/$100 under E-5.		$150/individual or $300/family.	
Monthly Premium	$54.35/individual or $192.89/family		$419.72/individual or $1,024.43/family	
Annual Out-of-Pocket Limit	$1,000/family per fiscal year		$3,000/family per fiscal year	
Fees for Medical Services	in-network	out of network	in-network	out of network
Civilian Outpatient Visit	15% of negotiated rate	20% of negotiated rate	20% of allowable charge	25% of allowable charge
Emergency Room Visit	15% of negotiated rate	20% of negotiated rate	20% of allowable charge	25% of allowable charge
Hospitalization	Greater of $17.05/day or $25	Greater of $17.05/day or $25	Lesser of $250/day or 25% of billed charges for institutional services, plus 20% of separately billed services	Lesser of $708/day or 25% of billed charges for institutional services, plus 25% of separately billed services
Civilian Inpatient Behavioral Health	Greater of $20/day or $25	Greater of $20/day or $25	20% of total charge plus 20% of allowable charge for separately billed professional services	High-Volume Hospital: 25% of hospital-specific per diem Low-Volume Hospital: Lesser of $208 per day or 25% of billed charges

Source: TRICARE web site. Beneficiary costs current as of October 1, 2012.
For out-of-pocket limits, please see http://www.tricare.mil/mybenefit/home/Costs/HealthPlanCosts
For full beneficiary cost tables for TRICARE Reserve Select, please see http://www.tricare.mil/mybenefit/home/Costs/HealthPlanCosts/TRICAREReserveSelect?.
For full beneficiary cost tables for TRICARE Retired Reserve, please see http://www.tricare.mil/mybenefit/home/Costs/HealthPlanCosts/TRICARERetiredReserve?

Table 4. Selected TRICARE Fees for TRICARE Young Adult

	Prime		Standard	
	Children of Active Duty Service Members and Sponsors Using TRICARE Reserve Select		All Others including Children of Sponsors Using TRICARE Retired Reserve	
Annual Deductible	None		$150/individual or $300/family	
Monthly Premium	$201		$176	
Annual Out-of-Pocket Limit	$3,000/ family per fiscal year		$3,000/family per fiscal year	
Fees for Medical Services	**in-network**	**out of network**	**in-network**	**out of network**
Civilian Outpatient Visit	$12/visit	20% of allowable charge	20% of negotiated rate	25% of allowable charge
Emergency Room Visit	$30/visit	20% of allowable charge	20% of negotiated rate	25% of allowable charge
Hospitalization	Greater of $11/day or $25	Greater of $17.05/day or $25	Lesser of $250/day or 25% of billed charges for institutional services, plus 20% of separately billed services	Lesser of $708/day or 25% of billed charges for institutional services, plus 25% of separately billed services
Civilian Inpatient Behavioral Health	$40/day, no charge for separately billed professional services	Greater of $20/day or $25	20% of total charge plus 20% of allowable charge for separately billed professional services	High-Volume Hospital: 25% of hospital-specific per diem Low-Volume Hospital: Lesser of $208 per day or 25% of billed charges

Source: TRICARE web site. Beneficiary costs current as of October 1, 2012.

For out-of-pocket limits, please see http://www.tricare.mil/mybenefit/home/Costs/ HealthPlanCosts

For full beneficiary cost tables for TRICARE Young Adult Prime, please see http://www.tricare.mil/mybenefit/home/Costs/ HealthPlanCosts/TRICAREYoungAdult/PrimeOption

For full beneficiary cost tables for TRICARE Young Adult Standard, please see http://www.tricare.mil/mybenefit/home/Costs/ HealthPlanCosts/TRICAREYoungAdult/StandardOption?

Table 5. TRICARE for Life Fees and Payment Structure

Type of Medical Service	What Medicare Pays	What TRICARE for Life Pays	What Beneficiary Pays
If covered by TRICARE and Medicare	Medicare's authorized amount	Remainder	$0
If covered by Medicare but not TRICARE	Medicare's authorized amount	$0	Medicare deductible and cost-share
If covered by TRICARE but not Medicare	$0	TRICARE's authorized amount	TRICARE deductible and cost-share
If not covered by TRICARE or Medicare	$0	$0	Full amount

Source: TRICARE, "TRICARE Choices at a Glance," May 2012. http://www. humana-military.com/library/pdf/cost-summary.pdf

7. What Is the DOD Pharmacy Benefit?

Those with access to military treatment facilities and those who are enrolled in TRICARE Prime receive prescribed pharmaceuticals free of charge. In accordance with the provisions of the FY2001 Defense Authorization Act (P.L. 106-398), effective April 1, 2001, retirees have access to DOD's National Mail Order Pharmacy and retail pharmacies in addition to pharmacies in military treatment facilities. Beneficiaries who turned 65 prior to April 1, 2001, qualify for the benefit whether or not they purchased Medicare Part B; beneficiaries who attain the age of 65 on or after April 1, 2001, must be enrolled in Medicare Part B to receive the pharmacy benefit. (There are deductibles for use of non-network pharmacies and co-payments for pharmaceuticals received from the National Mail Order Pharmacy and from retail pharmacies.)

Military pharmacies do not necessarily carry every pharmaceutical available; thus, even some with access to military facilities must have certain prescriptions filled in civilian pharmacies; for these prescriptions beneficiaries can be reimbursed through TRICARE.

In October 1997, DOD implemented the National Mail Order Pharmacy (subsequently known as the TRICARE Mail Order Pharmacy) that allows beneficiaries to obtain some pharmaceuticals by mail with small handling charges. The mail order program is designed to fill long-term prescriptions to treat conditions such as high blood pressure, asthma, or diabetes; it does not include medications that require immediate attention such as some antibiotics. Prescriptions filled by the TRICARE Mail Order Pharmacy in fiscal year 2012 cost $0 for a 90-day supply of a generic medication, $9 for a 90-day supply of a brand-name formulary medication, and $25 for a 90-day supply of a non-formulary medication.[7]

In 2004 DOD, in response to guidance in the FY2000 Defense Authorization Act (P.L. 106-65, Section 701), established a uniform formulary to discourage use of expensive pharmaceuticals when others are medically appropriate. Regulations to this effect were published in the Federal Register on April 1, 2004 (vol. 69, pp. 17035-17052). Section 703 of the FY2008 National Defense Authorization (P.L. 110-181) made pharmaceuticals purchased by TRICARE beneficiaries through retail pharmacies subject to federal pricing schedules. Prescriptions filled by a retail network pharmacy in fiscal year 2012 cost $5 for a 30-day supply of a generic medication, $12 for a 30-day supply of a brand-name formulary medication, and $25 for a 30-day supply of a non-formulary medication.[8]

The Secretary of Defense is authorized to set and adjust copayment requirements for the pharmacy program under 10 U.S.C. 1074g.

8. Who Is Eligible to Receive Care?

Eligibility for TRICARE is determined by the uniformed services and reported to the Defense Enrollment Eligibility Reporting System (DEERS). All eligible beneficiaries must have their eligibility status recorded in DEERS.

TRICARE beneficiaries can be divided into two main categories: sponsors and dependents. Sponsors are usually active duty service members, National Guard/Reserve members or retired service members. "Sponsor" refers to the person who is serving or who has served on active duty or in the National Guard or Reserves. "Dependent" is defined at 10 U.S.C. 1072 and includes a variety of relationships, for example, spouses, children, certain unremarried former spouses, etc.

Figure 2 below illustrates the major categories of eligible beneficiaries.

9. How Are Priorities for Care in Military Medical Facilities Assigned?

Active duty personnel, military retirees, and their respective dependents are not afforded equal access to care in military medical facilities. Active duty personnel receive top priority access and are "entitled" to health care in a military medical facility (10 U.S.C. 1074).

According to 10 U.S.C. 1076, dependents of active duty personnel are "entitled, upon request, to medical and dental care" on a space-available basis at a military medical facility. Title 10 U.S.C. 1074 states that "a member or former member of the uniformed services who is entitled to retired or retainer pay ... may, upon request, be given medical and dental care in any facility of the uniformed service" on a space-available basis.

This language entitles active duty dependents to medical and dental care subject to space-available limitations. No such entitlement or "right" is provided to retirees or their dependents. Instead, retirees and their dependents may be given medical and dental care, subject to the same space-available limitations. This language gives active duty personnel and their dependents priority in receiving medical and dental care at any facility of the uniformed services over military members entitled to receive retired pay and their dependents. The policy of providing active duty dependents priority over retirees in the receipt of medical and dental care in any facility of the uniformed services has existed in law since at least September 2, 1958 (P.L. 85-861).

Since the establishment of TRICARE and pursuant to the Defense Authorization Act of FY1996 (P.L. 104-106), DOD has established the following basic priorities (with certain special provisions):

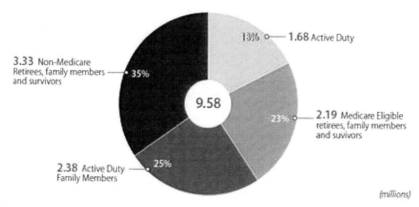

Source: The President's Budget for FY2013, Appendix, "Department of Defense – Military Programs," p. 271. Adapted by CRS.

Figure 2. Military Health System Eligible Beneficiaries (millions).

Priority 1: Active-duty service members;
Priority 2: Active-duty family members who are enrolled in TRICARE Prime;
Priority 3: Retirees, their family members and survivors who are enrolled in TRICARE Prime;
Priority 4: Active-duty family members who are not enrolled in TRICARE Prime;
Priority 5: All other eligible persons.

The priority is given to active duty dependents to help them obtain care easily, and thus make it possible for active duty members to perform their military service without worrying about health care for their dependents. This is particularly important for active duty personnel who may be assigned overseas or aboard ship and separated from their dependents. As retirees are not subject to such imposed separations, they are considered to be in a better position to see that their dependents receive care, if care cannot be provided in a military facility. Thus, the role of health care delivery recognizes the unique needs of the military mission. The role of health care in the military is qualitatively different, and, therefore, not necessarily comparable to the civilian sector.

The benefits available to service members or retirees, which require comparatively little or no contributions from the beneficiaries themselves, are considered by some to be a more generous benefit package than is available to civil servants or to most people in the private sector. Retirees may also be eligible to receive medical care at Department of Veterans Affairs (VA) medical facilities.[9]

10. What Are the Long-Term Trends in Defense Health Costs?

Even as the number of active duty personnel in DOD declines over the next few years, costs associated with the military health system are expected to grow. Total military health system costs (excluding TRICARE for Life) increased between FY 2009 and FY 2011 for inpatient and outpatient services but declined for prescription drugs, due to the FY2008 NDAA requirement that the TRICARE retail pharmacy program be subject to the same pricing standards as other federal agencies.

DOD's FY2013 appropriations request for the Defense Health Program and the Medical Eligible Retiree Health Fund is approximately 7.4% of DOD's total FY2013 appropriations request.[10] The Congressional Budget Office (CBO) projects that the cost of the military health care system will grow from $51 billion in FY2013 (higher than DOD's FY2013 budget request of $47 billion) to $65 billion by FY2017 and $95 billion by FY2030.[11] Over the FYDP period from FY2013 – FY2017, CBO's projection has average annual growth of 6.0%, compared with 2.6% in DOD's projection. Over the entire 2013–2030 period, CBO estimates the real (inflation-adjusted) growth rates in cost per user in the military health system would average 5.5% per year for pharmaceuticals, 4.7% for purchased care and contracts, and 3.3% for direct care and administration. Overall, DOD forecasts expect Defense Health Program costs to increase by 3.4% in FY2014, 3.35% in FY2015, 3.6% in FY2016 and 3.9% in FY2017, in constant FY2013 dollars.[12]

This cost growth stems in part from general inflation in the cost of health care, as well as an increasing percentage of care being provided to retirees and their dependents. DOD estimates that care provided to retirees and their dependents will make up over 65% of DOD health care costs by 2015, up from 43% in 1999.[13] A recent CBO analysis concludes that this increasing proportion of retirees participating in TRICARE is driven by "low out-of-pocket expenses for TRICARE beneficiaries (many of whose copayments, deductibles, and maximum annual out-of-pocket payments have remained unchanged or have decreased since the mid-1990s), combined with increased costs of alternative sources of health insurance coverage."[14] In addition, CBO found that TRICARE beneficiaries use both inpatient and outpatient care at rates significantly higher than people with other insurance, due to low out-of-pocket costs and other factors.

DOD proposed new fees and cost-sharing increases for retiree TRICARE plans in their FY2013 budget submission. The new fee proposals were generally based on recommendations by the 2007 Task Force on the Future of Military Health Care. This Congressionally-created Task Force found that, "because costs borne by retirees under age 65 have been fixed in dollar terms since 1996, when TRICARE was being established, the portion of medical care costs assumed by these military retirees has declined by a factor of 2-3."[15] Overall, "military health care premiums paid by individual military retirees under age 65 utilizing DOD's most popular plan (TRICARE Prime) have fallen from 11% to 4 %" of total health care costs.[16] These proposed cost-sharing increases and new fees would require new legislation.

11. How Does the Patient Protection and Affordable Care Act Affect TRICARE?

In general, the Patient Protection and Affordable Care Act (PPACA)(P.L. 111-148) does not directly affect TRICARE administration, health care benefits, eligibility, or cost to beneficiaries.[17]

Section 3110 of the PPACA does open a special Medicare Part B enrollment window to enable certain individuals to gain coverage under the TRICARE for Life program.[18] The PPACA also waives the Medicare Part B late enrollment penalty during the 12-month special enrollment period (SEP) for military retirees, their spouses (including widows/widowers), and dependent children who are otherwise eligible for TRICARE and are entitled to Medicare Part A based on disability or end-stage renal disease, but have declined Part B. The Secretary of Defense is required to identify and notify individuals of their eligibility for the SEP; the Secretary of Health and Human Services (HHS) and the Commissioner for Social Security must support these efforts. Section 3110 of the PPACA was amended by the Medicare and Medicaid Extenders Act of 2010[19] to clarify that Section 3110 applies to Medicare Part B elections made on or after the date of enactment of the PPACA, which was on March 23, 2010.

12. How Are Private Health Care Providers Paid?

By law (P.L. 102-396) and Federal Regulation (32 CFR 199.14), health care providers treating TRICARE patients cannot bill for more than 115% of charges authorized by a DOD fee schedule. In some geographic areas, providers have been unwilling to accept TRICARE patients because of the limits on fees that can be charged. DOD has authority to grant exceptions. Statutes (10 U.S.C. 1079) also require that payment levels for health care services provided under TRICARE be aligned with Medicare's fee schedule "to the extent practicable." Over 90% of TRICARE payment levels are now equivalent to those authorized by Medicare, about 10% are higher, and steps are being taken to adjust some to Medicare levels.

For institutional providers of outpatient services, TRICARE recently published a final regulation[20] that became effective on May 1, 2009, implementing the TRICARE outpatient prospective payment system (OPPS). Under 10 U.S.C. 1079(h) and 1079(j)(2), DOD is required to use Medicare's reimbursement payment system for hospital outpatient services to the extent practicable. Under the OPPS, hospital outpatient services are paid on a rate-per-service basis that varies according to the Ambulatory Payment Classification (APC) group to which the services are assigned. Group services identified by Health Care Procedure Coding System (HCPCS) codes and descriptors within APC groups are the basis for setting payment rates under the hospital OPPS. To receive TRICARE reimbursement under the OPPS, providers must follow all Medicare specific coding requirements, except in those instances where the TRICARE Management Activity (TMA) develops specific APCs for those services that are unique to the TRICARE beneficiary population. For inpatient services, TMA regularly publishes reimbursement schedules through the Federal Register.

13. What Is the Relationship of DOD Health Care to Medicare?

TRICARE and Medicare Payments to Providers and the Sustainable Growth Rate

Under 10 U.S.C. 1079, TRICARE is required to pay healthcare providers "to the extent practicable in accordance with the same reimbursement rules as apply to payments" under Medicare. This requirement was added by Section 731 of the National Defense Authorization Act for Fiscal Year 1996 (P.L. 104-106, February 10, 1996).

The Sustainable Growth Rate (SGR) is the statutory method for determining the annual updates to the Medicare physician fee schedule, created in the Budget Control Act of 1997 (see Section 1848 of the Social Security Act codified at 42 U.S.C. 1395w–4.) Under the SGR formula, if [Medicare] expenditures over a period are less than the cumulative spending target for the period, the annual update [to the provider fee schedule] is increased. However, if spending exceeds the cumulative spending target over a certain period, future updates are reduced to bring spending back in line with the target." In other words, if Medicare costs are greater than expected, the provider fees are reduced to bring overall Medicare expenditures down towards expected levels.

Each year since 2002, the sustainable growth rate (SGR) system, has produced a formula result (technically referred to as a "conversion factor") that would reduce reimbursement rates. With the exception of 2002, when a 4.8% decrease was applied, Congress has persistently declined to apply the SGR formula-driven reductions to provider fee rates through a series of temporary postponements known as "doc fixes."

Most recently, when President Obama signed the Middle Class Tax Relief and Job Creation Act of 2012 (P.L. 112-96) on February 22, 2012, the implementation of the SGR formula-driven reimbursement rates was again delayed until January 1, 2013. Absent legislation, the Medicare reimbursement rate reduction on January 1, 2013 has been estimated by the Department of Health and Human Services to be 27.4%.[21]

Although the law requires TRICARE reimbursement rates to be equal to Medicare rates "to the extent practicable," it does permit TRICARE to make exceptions to ensure an adequate network of providers or to eliminate a situation of severely impaired access to care.

Medicare and TRICARE for Life

Active duty military personnel have been fully covered by Social Security and have paid Social Security taxes since January 1, 1957. In 1965, Congress created Medicare under Title XVIII of the Social Security Act to provide health insurance to people age 65 and older, regardless of income or medical history. Social Security coverage includes eligibility for health care coverage under Medicare at age 65.

In establishing CHAMPUS in 1966, it was the legislative intent of the Congress that retired members of the uniformed services and their eligible dependents be provided with medical care after they retire from the military, usually between their late-30s and mid-40s. However, Congress did not intend that CHAMPUS should replace Medicare as a supplemental benefit to military health care. For this reason, retirees became ineligible to receive CHAMPUS benefits when, at age 65, they become eligible for Medicare.

Many argued that the structure was inherently unfair because retirees lost TRICARE/CHAMPUS benefits at the stage in life when they were increasingly likely to need them. It was argued that military personnel had been promised free medical care for life, not just until age 65. After considerable debate over various options for ensuring medical care to retired beneficiaries, Congress in the FY2001 Defense Authorization Act (P.L. 106-259) provided that, beginning October 1, 2001, TRICARE pays out-of-pocket costs for services provided under Medicare for beneficiaries over age 64 if they are enrolled in Medicare Part B. This benefit is known as TRICARE for Life (TFL). Disabled persons under 65 who are entitled to Medicare may continue to receive CHAMPUS benefits as a second payer to Medicare Parts A and B (with some restrictions).

The requirement for enrollment in Medicare Part B, which had typical premiums of $99.40 per month in 2012[22], is a source of concern to some beneficiaries, especially those who did not enroll in Part B when they became 65 and thus must pay significant penalties. Some argue that this requirement is unfair since Part B enrollment was not originally a prerequisite for access to any DOD medical care. On the other hand, waiving the penalty for military retirees could be considered unfair to other Medicare-users who did not enroll in Part B upon turning 65. The Medicare Prescription Drug, Improvement, and Modernization Act (P.L. 108-173), passed in December 2003, waived penalties for military retirees in certain circumstances during an open season in 2004.[23]

14. What Medical Benefits Are Available to Reservists?

Reservists and National Guardsmen (members of the "Reserve Component") who are serving on active duty have the same medical benefits as regular military personnel. Reserve personnel while on active duty for training and during weekly or monthly drills also are covered for illnesses incurred while on training or traveling to or from their duty station. In recent years, especially as members of the Reserve Component have had a larger role in combat operations overseas, Congress has broadened the medical benefits for Reservists. Those who have been notified that they are to be activated are now covered by TRICARE up to 90 days before reporting. Reservists who have served more than 30 days after having been called up for active duty in a contingency are eligible for 180 days of TRICARE coverage after the end of their service under the Transitional Assistance Management Program (TAMP). In addition, in 2004 Congress authorized (in P.L. 108-375, Section 701) the TRICARE Reserve Select (TRS) program for Reserve Component members called to active duty, under Title 10, in support of a contingency operation after September 11, 2001. To be eligible for TRS, reservists must agree to stay in the Reserves for one or more years and must pay monthly premiums (in 2012, $54.35 for individual coverage, $192.89 for member and family coverage).

15. Have Military Personnel been Promised Free Medical Care for Life?

Some military personnel and former military personnel maintain that they and their dependents were promised "free medical care for life" at the time of their enlistment. Such promises may have been made by military recruiters and in recruiting brochures; however, if they were made, they were not based upon laws or official regulations which provide only for access to military medical facilities for non-active duty personnel if space is available as described above. Space was not always available and TRICARE options could involve significant costs to beneficiaries.

Rear Admiral Harold M. Koenig, the Deputy Assistant Secretary of Defense for Health Affairs, testified in May 1993: "We have a medical care program for life for our beneficiaries, and it is pretty well defined in the law. That easily gets interpreted to, or reinterpreted into, free medical care for the rest of your life.

That is a pretty easy transition for people to make in their thinking, and it is pervasive. We [DOD] spend an incredible amount of effort trying to re-educate people [that] that is not their benefit."[24]

Dr. Stephen C. Joseph, Assistant Secretary of Defense for Health Affairs in April 1998, however, argued that because retirees believe they have had a promise of free care, the government did have an obligation. Joseph did not specify the precise extent of the obligation.

The FY1998 Defense Authorization Act (P.L. 105-85) included (in Section 752) a finding that "many retired military personnel believe that they were promised lifetime health care in exchange for 20 or more years of service," and expressed the sense of Congress that "the United States has incurred a moral obligation to provide health care to members and [retired] members of the Armed Services." Further, it is necessary "to provide quality, affordable care to such retirees."

16. What Is the Congressionally Directed Medical Research Program?

Many different entities within the Department of Defense request appropriations for and are funded to conduct a wide range of medical research. Over the last 17 years, Congress has supplemented the DOD appropriations to include additional unrequested funding for specific medical research funding. In 1992, Congress appropriated $25M for breast cancer research to be managed by DOD's U.S. Army Medical Research and Materiel Command (USAMRMC).

The following year, Congress appropriated $210M to the DOD for extramural, peer-reviewed breast cancer research.

Following this, DOD established the Congressionally Directed Medical Research Programs (CDMRP), within USAMRMC. The program now manages congressionally-directed appropriations totaling $6 billion through fiscal year 2010 for research on breast, prostate, and ovarian cancers; neurofibromatosis; military health; chronic myelogenous leukemia; tuberous sclerosis complex; autism; psychological health and traumatic brain injury; amyotrophic lateral sclerosis; Gulf War Illness; deployment-related health research; and other health concerns.[25]

This additional, unrequested funding, now appears in the Defense Health Program RDT&E appropriation. Conference report language usually includes a table instructing the Department of Defense on how to allocate the additional funding to specific diseases and research areas.

This guidance is not considered to be an earmark because the funding is used for peer-reviewed, competitively awarded research grants.

Table 6, below, depicts appropriations for selected CDMRP programs.

Table 6. Appropriation Levels by Fiscal Year (FY) for Selected CDMR Programs, FY2007 – FY2012
(in millions of current dollars)

	FY 2007a	FY 2008b	FY 2009c	FY2010d	FY2011e	FY2012f
Amyotrophic Lateral Sclerosis	5	0	5	7.5	8	6.4
Autism	7.5	6.4	8	8	6.4	5.1
Bone Marrow Failure	0	0	5	3.75	4	3.2
Breast Cancer/Breast Cancer Research	127.5	138	150	150	150	120
Genetic Studies of Food Allergies	0	0	2.5	1.875	0	0
Gulf War Illness	0	10	8	8	8	10
Lung Cancer	0	0	20	15	12.8	10.2
Multiple Sclerosis	0	0	5	4.5	4.8	3.8
Neurofibromatosis	10	8	10	13.75	16	0
Ovarian Cancer	10	10	20	18.75	20	16
Peer-Reviewed Cancer	0	0	16	15	16	12.8
Peer-Reviewed Medical	0	0	50	50	50	50

Table 6. (Continued)

	FY 2007a	FY 2008b	FY 2009c	FY2010d	FY2011e	FY2012f
Peer-Reviewed Orthopedic	0	0	51	22.5	24	30
Post-Traumatic Stress Disorder (PTSD)	151	0	0	0	0	0
Prostate Cancer	80	80	80	80	80	80
Psychological Health/Traumatic Brain Injury	150	0	165	120	100	135.5
Spinal Cord Injury	0	0	35	11.25	12	9.6
Tuberous Sclerosis	0	4	6	6	6.4	5.1

Source: Congressionally Directed Medical Research Program, Annual Reports FY2007 – FY2012, Recommendations accompanying the Defense Appropriations Acts.

Notes:

a. Funds appropriated by P.L. 110-5 (see H.Rept. 109-676 to H.R. 5631, September 25, 2006, pages 248-250). http://www.gpo.gov/fdsys/pkg/CRPT-109hrpt676/pdf/CRPT-109hrpt676.pdf

b. Funds appropriated by P.L. 110-116. See *Congressional Record*, November 6, 2007, p. H13119.

c. Funds appropriated by Division C of P.L. 110-329. *See Congressional Record*, September 24, 2008, pp. H9725 – H9726.

d. Funds appropriated by P.L. 111-117. See Congressional Record, December 16, 2009, p. H15319 – H15320. http://www.gpo.gov/fdsys/pkg/CREC-2009-12-16/pdf/CREC-2009-12-16-pt1-PgH15007-2.pdf#page=314

e. Funds appropriated by P.L. 112-10. See House Rules Committee' tables accompanying H.R. 1473, pp. 53-54. http://rules.house.gov/Media/file/FY11-Defense-Department-Base-tables.pdf

f. Funds appropriated by P.L. 112-74 (H.R. 2055). See House Rules Committee's tables accompanying H.R. 2055, 92A, p. 282. http://rules.house.gov/Media/file/PDF_112_1/legislativetext/H.R. 2055crSOM/psConference%20Div%20A%20-%20SOM%20OCR.pdf

The CDMRP web site (http://cdmrp.army.mil/) also provides specific descriptions and funding histories of the different research programs.

17. Other Frequently Asked Questions

Does TRICARE Cover Abortion?

10 U.S.C. 1093 provides that "Funds available to the Department of Defense may not be used to perform abortions except where the life of the mother would be endangered if the fetus were carried to term."

Does DOD Use Animals in Medical Research or Training?

Yes. DOD policy is that live animals will not be used for training and education except where, after exhaustive analysis, no alternatives are available. Currently approved uses include pre-deployment training for medical personnel and include infant intubation (ferrets); microsurgery (rodents); and combat trauma training (goats and swine).

End Notes

[1] Department of Defense, *Task Force on the Future of Military Health Care*, December 2007, pp. 113-116.

[2] Department of Defense, *FY 2013 Budget Request Overview*, February 2012, pp. 5-2, Figure 5-1. http://comptroller.defense.gov/defbudget/fy2013/FY2013_Budget_Request_Overview_Boo k.pdf

[3] Department of Defense, *Fiscal Year 2011 Medicare-Eligible Retiree Health Care Fun Audited Financial Statements*, November 7, 2011, p. 5, http://comptroller.defense.gov/cfs/fy2011/ 12_Medicare_Eligible_Retiree_Health_Care_Fund/Fiscal_Year_2011_Medicare_Eligible_ Retiree_Health_Care_Fund_Financial_Statements_and_Notes.pdf.

[4] P.L. 84-569.

[5] P.L 89-614.

[6] 10 U.S.C. §1086(d).

[7] TRICARE Pharmacy Benefit Handbook, Figure 5.1, p. 22. http://www.tricare.mil/mybenefit/ Download/Forms/Pharmacy_HBK.pdf

[8] TRICARE Pharmacy Benefit Handbook, Figure 5.1, p. 22. http://www.tricare.mil/mybenefit/ Download/Forms/Pharmacy_HBK.pdf

[9] See CRS Report RL32975, *Veterans' Medical Care: FY2006 Appropriations*, by Sidath Viranga Panangala.

[10] Comptroller, Department of Defense. National Defense Budget Estimates for FY2013, March 2012. Table 3-1, Reconciliation of Authorization, Appropriation, TOA and BA, by Program, by Appropriation. pp. 36-44. http://comptroller.defense.gov/defbudget/fy2013/ FY13_Green_Book.pdf

[11] Congressional Budget Office, *Long Term Implications of the 2013 Future Years Defense Program*, p. 21, http://www.cbo.gov/sites/default/files/cbofiles/attachments/07-11-12-FYDP_forPosting_0.pdf.

[12] Comptroller, Department of Defense. *National Defense Budget Estimates for FY2013*, March 2012. Table 5-5, Department of Defense Deflators – TOA. p. 60. http://comptroller.defense. gov/defbudget/fy2013/FY13_Green_Book.pdf

[13] Department of Defense, Report of The Tenth Quadrennial Review of Military Compensation: Volume II Deferred and Noncash Compensation, July 2008, p. 45.

[14] Congressional Budget Office, *Long Term Implications of the 2013 Future Years Defense Program*, p. 21, http://www.cbo.gov/sites/default/files/cbofiles/attachments/07-11-12-FYDP _ forPosting_0.pdf. p. 22.

[15] Department of Defense, subcommittee of the Defense Health Board, "Report of the Task Force on the Future of Military Health Care," December 2007, p. ES10. http://www.dcoe.health.mil/Content/Navigation/Documents/103-06-2-Home-Task_Force_FINAL_REPORT _122007.pdf

[16] Department of Defense, subcommittee of the Defense Health Board, "Report of the Task Force on the Future of Military Health Care," December 2007, p. 92. http://www.dcoe.health.mil/Content/Navigation/Documents/103-06-2-Home-Task_Force_FINAL_REPORT_122007.pdf

[17] CRS Report R41198, *TRICARE and VA Health Care: Impact of the Patient Protection and Affordable Care Act (ACA)*, by Sidath Viranga Panangala and Don J. Jansen.

[18] §3110 of PPACA, P.L. 111-148.

[19] §201, P.L. 111-309.

[20] Department of Defense, "TRICARE: Outpatient Hospital Prospective Payment System (OPPS); Delay of Effective Date and Additional Opportunity for Public Comment," 74 *Federal Register* 6228, February 6, 2009.

[21] Centers for Medicare and Medicaid Services, "Estimated Sustainable Growth Rate and Conversion Factor, for Medicare Payments to Physicians in 2012," Table 5, p. 7. http://www.cms.gov/Medicare/Medicare-Fee-for-Service-Payment/SustainableGRatesConFact/downloads/sgr2012f.pdf

[22] Department of Health and Human Services, "Medicare Part B premiums for 2012 lower than projected," press release, 2011, http://www.hhs.gov/news/press/2011pres/10/20111027a.html.

[23] See CRS Report RS21731, *Medicare: Part B Premium Penalty*, by Jennifer O'Sullivan.

[24] U.S. Congress, House of Representatives, Committee on Armed Services, Military Forces and Personnel Subcommittee, 103rd Congress, 1st session, *National Defense Authorization Act for Fiscal Year 1994—H.R. 2401 and Oversight of Previously Authorized Programs*, Hearings, H.A.S.C. No. 103-13, April 27, 28, May 10, 11, and 13, 1993, p. 505.

[25] Department of Defense, Congressionally Directed Medical Research Program: FY 2008 Annual Report, September 30, 2008, pp. 1-2, http://cdmrp.army.mil/annreports/2008 annrep/ default.htm.

In: Military Health Care
Editor: Brian M. Gagliardi

ISBN: 978-1-62417-339-4
© 2013 Nova Science Publishers, Inc.

Chapter 2

TRICARE AND VA HEALTH CARE: IMPACT OF THE PATIENT PROTECTION AND AFFORDABLE CARE ACT (ACA)*

Sidath Viranga Panangala and Don J. Jansen

SUMMARY

The 111th Congress passed, and the President signed into law, the Patient Protection and Affordable Care Act (P.L. 111-148; ACA), as amended by the Health Care and Education Reconciliation Act of 2010 (P.L. 111-152; HCERA), and hereafter referred to as ACA. In general, ACA did not make any significant changes to the Department of Defense (DOD) TRICARE program or to the Department of Veterans Affairs (VA) health care system. However, many have sought clarification as to whether certain provisions in ACA, such as a mandate for most individuals to have health insurance, or extending dependant coverage up to age 26, would apply to TRICARE and VA health care beneficiaries.

To address some of these concerns, Congress has introduced and/or enacted legislation. The TRICARE Affirmation Act (H.R. 4887; P.L. 111-159), signed into law on April 26, 2010, affirms that TRICARE satisfies the minimum acceptable coverage requirement in ACA. Similarly, P.L. 111-173,

---

* This is an edited, reformatted and augmented version of the Congressional Research Service Publication, CRS Report for Congress R41198, dated January 27, 2012.

signed into law on May 27, 2010, clarifies that the Civilian Health and Medical Program of the Department of Veterans Affairs (CHAMPVA), Spina Bifida Health Care Program, and the Children of Women Vietnam Veterans Health Care Program meet the "minimum essential coverage" requirement under ACA. TRICARE coverage of children was extended to age 26 by the Ike Skelton National Defense Authorization Act for Fiscal Year 2011 (P.L. 111-383).

ACA requires that if a health insurance plan provides for dependent coverage of children, the plan must continue to make such coverage available for an adult child until age 26. This requirement relating to coverage of adult children will take effect for the plan years beginning on or after September 23, 2010. Under ACA, both married and unmarried children will qualify for this coverage. The authorizing statute for CHAMPVA currently does not conform to this ACA requirement. Furthermore, although the TRICARE authorizing statute has been amended to provide for coverage of children until age 26, the coverage provided by the new legislation differs from that required by ACA in some important ways. To address the CHAMPVA situation, the CHAMPVA Children's Protection Act of 2011 (H.R. 115) has been introduced in the 112th Congress, although it has seen no action so far.

This report addresses key questions concerning how ACA affects TRICARE and VA health care.

INTRODUCTION

On March 23, 2010, President Obama signed the Patient Protection and Affordable Care Act (P.L. 111-148, ACA). On March 30, 2010, ACA was amended by P.L. 111-152, the Health Care and Education Reconciliation Act of 2010 (HCERA). Throughout this report, this amended version is referred to as ACA. This health reform legislation touched on many aspects of the nation's health care delivery and financing systems. However, in general, ACA did not make any significant changes to the Department of Defense (DOD) TRICARE program or to the Department of Veterans Affairs (VA) health care system.

Among its numerous provisions, ACA (when fully implemented in 2014) will require most individuals, large employers, and health plans to meet certain coverage requirements. Beginning in 2014, ACA includes a mandate for most individuals to have health insurance,[1] or potentially pay a penalty for noncompliance.[2] Individuals will be required to maintain minimum essential coverage for themselves and their dependents. Those who do not meet the mandate will be required to pay a penalty for each month of noncompliance. Under ACA, private health insurance provisions that take effect prior to 2014 (including some this year) include the following: ending lifetime and unreasonable annual limits on benefits, prohibiting rescissions of health insurance policies, requiring coverage of preventive services and immunizations, extending dependant coverage up to age 26, capping insurance companies' nonmedical administrative expenditures, guaranteeing coverage for preexisting health conditions for enrollees under age 19, and providing assistance for those who are uninsured because of a preexisting condition. Furthermore, ACA raises revenues to pay for expanded health insurance coverage by imposing excise taxes and fees on industries in the health care sector, limiting tax-advantaged health accounts, and increasing the Medicare payroll tax on upper-income households and adding an additional tax on net investment income on upper-income households.[3]

Since the enactment of ACA, concerns have been raised by veterans and Veterans Service Organizations (VSOs) on how the new law would affect TRICARE beneficiaries, as well as veterans and certain dependents receiving care through the VA health care system.[4] Moreover, many have sought clarification as to whether certain provisions in ACA, such as a mandate for most individuals to have health insurance, or extending dependant coverage up to age 26, would apply to TRICARE and VA health care beneficiaries.[5] Although the Obama Administration issued statements assuring that the two health care systems would not be negatively affected, some veterans groups have been demanding statutory clarification.[6] To address some of these concerns, Congress has introduced and/or enacted legislation. This report, one of a series of CRS products on ACA, addresses key questions concerning the impact of enactment of the ACA on the TRICARE and VA health care programs. To provide some context to this discussion, the report begins with a brief overview of the two health care systems and eligibility for care under each system.

BACKGROUND

TRICARE[7]

The Department of Defense (DOD) administers health care services through a program known as TRICARE to over 9 million eligible beneficiaries that include active duty uniformed personnel and their dependents, eligible members of the Reserve Component and their dependents, and uniformed services retirees and their dependents and survivors. TRICARE provides health care services through both military and nonmilitary hospitals, clinics, and other providers. TRICARE is administered on a regional basis by the TRICARE Management Activity, which uses a regional managed care support contractor to develop networks of civilian providers and process beneficiary claims in each of its North, South, and West regions. TRICARE has three basic options for non-Medicare eligible beneficiaries: TRICARE Prime, which is a managed care option that relies primarily upon military providers and treatment facilities; a fee-for-service option known as TRICARE Standard; and a preferred-provider option known as TRICARE Extra. Individuals who are eligible for Medicare and otherwise eligible for TRICARE may enroll in Medicare Part B and receive "wrap-around" TRICARE coverage through the TRICARE for Life Program, which covers costs not paid by Medicare that would otherwise be incurred by the beneficiary.

The VA Health Care System and Eligibility for Care[8]

The Department of Veterans Affairs (VA), through the Veterans Health Administration (VHA), operates the nation's largest integrated direct health care delivery system.[9] While Medicare, Medicaid, and the Children's Health Insurance Program (CHIP) are also publicly funded programs, most health care services under these programs are delivered by private providers in private facilities. In contrast, the VA health care system could be categorized as a veteran-specific national health care system in the sense that the federal government owns the medical facilities and employs the health care providers.[10]

In general, eligibility for VA health care is based on veteran status,[11] presence of service-connected disabilities[12] or exposures,[13] income,[14] and/or other factors, such as status as a former prisoner of war or receipt of a Purple Heart.

The VHA also pays for care provided to veterans by private-sector providers on a fee basis under certain circumstances. Inpatient and outpatient care are also provided in the private sector to eligible dependents of veterans under the Civilian Health and Medical Program of the Department of Veterans Affairs (CHAMPVA; see discussion below). All enrolled veterans are offered a standard medical benefits package.[15]

Veterans do not pay premiums or enrollment fees. However, under current law most veterans are required to pay copayments for the treatment of nonservice-connected conditions.[16] It should be noted that those veterans who are rated 50% or more service-connected disabled and enrolled in the VA health care system do not pay copayments even for nonservice-connected care. Moreover, VA is required to collect reasonable charges for medical care or services (including prescription drugs) from a third-party insurer to the extent that the veteran or the provider of the care or services would be eligible to receive payment from a third-party insurer for a nonservice-connected disability for which the veteran is entitled to care (or the payment of expenses of care) under a health insurance plan.[17]

Civilian Health and Medical Program of the Department of Veterans Affairs (CHAMPVA)[18]

Unlike TRICARE, VA health care covers only a select group of dependents. In 1973, Congress established the Civilian Health and Medical Program of the Department of Veterans Affairs (CHAMPVA) as a means of providing health care services to dependents and survivors of certain veterans.[19] CHAMPVA primarily is a fee-for-service program that provides reimbursement for most medical care for certain eligible dependents and survivors of veterans rated permanently and totally disabled from a service-connected condition. CHAMPVA was designed to provide medical care in a manner similar to the care provided to certain eligible beneficiaries under the DOD TRICARE program. Eligibility for CHAMPVA requires inclusion in one of the following categories:[20]

- the individual is the spouse or child of a veteran who has been rated permanently and totally disabled for a service-connected disability;
- the individual is the surviving spouse or child of a veteran who died from a VA-rated service-connected disability;
- the individual is the surviving spouse or child of a veteran who was at the time of death rated permanently and totally disabled from a service-connected disability; or
- the individual is the surviving spouse or child of a military member who died on active duty, not due to misconduct (in most cases, these family members are eligible under TRICARE, not CHAMPVA).

QUESTIONS AND ANSWERS

How Does ACA Affect TRICARE?

In general, ACA does not affect TRICARE administration, health care benefits, eligibility, or cost to beneficiaries.

ACA does open a special Medicare Part B enrollment window to enable certain individuals to gain coverage under the TRICARE for Life program.[21] TRICARE was extended to Medicare-eligible military retirees, their Medicare-eligible spouses and dependent children, and Medicare-eligible widow/widowers by the Floyd D. Spence National Defense Authorization Act of 2001 (P.L. 106-398). This law established the TRICARE For Life (TFL) program, which acts as a secondary payer to Medicare and provides supplemental coverage to TRICARE-eligible beneficiaries who are entitled to Medicare Part A based on age, disability, or end-stage renal disease (ESRD). In order to participate in TFL, these TRICARE-eligible beneficiaries must enroll in and pay premiums for Medicare Part B. TRICARE-eligible beneficiaries who are entitled to Medicare Part A based on age, disability, or ESRD, but decline Part B, lose eligibility for TRICARE benefits.[22] In addition, individuals who choose not to enroll in Medicare Part B upon becoming eligible may elect to do so later during an annual enrollment period; however, the Medicare Part B late enrollment penalty would apply. ACA also waives the Medicare Part B late enrollment penalty during the 12-month special enrollment period (SEP) for military retirees, their spouses (including widows/widowers), and dependent children who are otherwise eligible for TRICARE and are entitled to Medicare Part A based on disability or ESRD, but have declined Part B. The Secretary of Defense is required to identify and notify individuals of their eligibility for the SEP; the Secretary of Health and Human Services (HHS) and the Commissioner for Social Security must support these efforts. This section was amended by the Medicare and Medicaid Extenders Act of 2010[23] to clarify that Section 3110 applies to Medicare Part B elections made on or after the date of enactment of ACA. This is the only provision in ACA that has an effect on beneficiary eligibility under the TRICARE program.

A 2011 Government Accountability Office report indicates that, overall, DOD expects to incur minimal costs to implement applicable ACA and HCERA provisions with which department officials have determined it is required to comply.[24]

How Does ACA Affect VA Health Care?

In general, ACA does not appear to affect current VA health care benefits, eligibility, or cost to beneficiaries.

However, ACA does contain several provisions related to the VA. Specifically, it includes a provision (§9011) that requires the VA to report to Congress on the effect to VA health care regarding the annual fee imposed by ACA on certain manufacturers and importers of branded prescription drugs, as well as the a new excise tax imposed on the sale of medical devices by manufacturers, producers, or importers (see question on medical devices below). Furthermore, it requires VA to participate in the Interagency Working Group on Health Care Quality (§3012), exempts the VA from a fee on all health insurers based on their market share (§4377), and provides VA access to the National Practitioner Data Bank without a charge (§6403).

Do TRICARE and VA Health Care Meet "Minimum Essential Coverage" Requirements?

It appears that TRICARE beneficiaries and veterans enrolled in the VA health care system would meet the minimum essential coverage requirements of ACA.

ACA requires certain individuals to maintain minimal essential health care coverage and provides a penalty for failure to maintain such coverage beginning in 2014. "Minimum essential coverage" is explicitly defined as coverage under VA Health Care; Medicare Part A; Medicaid; CHIP; the TRICARE for Life program; the Peace Corps program; an eligible employer-sponsored plan (as defined by ACA); a governmental plan (local, state, federal) including the Federal Employees Health Benefits Program (FEHBP) and any plan established by an Indian tribal government; any plan offered in the individual, small group, or large group market; a grandfathered health plan; and any other health benefits coverage, such as a state health benefits risk pool, as recognized by the HHS Secretary in coordination with the Treasury Secretary. The relevant definition[25] of "government plan" includes the TRICARE program beyond the TRICARE for Life program. However, because TRICARE is not explicitly listed as minimum essential coverage, some concern had been expressed by beneficiary groups that regular TRICARE coverage may not meet the requirement. The TRICARE Affirmation Act (H.R. 4887; P.L. 111-159), signed into law on April 26, 2010, amends the Internal Revenue Code to provide that TRICARE coverage satisfies the minimum essential coverage requirements as required by ACA. Likewise, P.L. 111-173, signed into law on May 27, 2010, clarifies that those enrolled in the VA health care system meet the minimum essential coverage requirement.

Will VA Coverage of Children with Spina Bifida and Certain Birth Defects Meet the "Minimum Essential Coverage" Requirement?

It was initially unclear whether the Spina Bifida Health Care Program (SBHCP) and the Children of Women Vietnam Veterans Health Care Program (CWVV) met the "minimum essential coverage" requirement under ACA. However, P.L. 111-173, signed into law on May 27, 2010, clarifies that CHAMPVA, SBHCP, and CWVV meet the minimum essential coverage requirement.

VA administers the Spina Bifida Health Care Program (SBHCP) for those biological children diagnosed with spina bifida of veterans who served in Vietnam, and of veterans who served in Korea during the period September 1, 1967, through August 31, 1971.[26] The program provides reimbursement for comprehensive medical care for those beneficiaries diagnosed with spina bifida except for conditions associated with spina bifida occulta. Similarly, VA administers the Children of Women Vietnam Veterans Health Care Program (CWVV). Under this program, VA reimburses for care of certain birth defects identified by the VA as resulting in permanent physical or mental disability of the biological child of a woman veteran who served in Vietnam between February 28, 1961, and May 7, 1975.[27]

Does ACA Require TRICARE to Provide Coverage to Dependent Children up to Age 26?

The ACA provision extending health insurance coverage to dependent children until age 26 did not extend to extend to TRICARE beneficiaries.

In general, eligibility for TRICARE is lost when either a dependent child turns 23 (if enrolled in an accredited school as a full-time student) or 21 if not enrolled. Section 1001 of ACA amends Part A of Title XXVII of the Public Health Service Act (PHSA) to add a new Section 2714 specifying that a group health plan and a health insurance issuer offering group or individual health insurance coverage that provides dependent coverage of children shall continue to make such coverage available for a until the dependent child turns 26 years of age. However, the provisions of title XXVII of the PHSA do not appear to apply to TRICARE.[28]

Coverage under the TRICARE program is governed by Chapter 55 of Title 10, *United States Code*. Under 10 U.S.C. §1072(2)(D), the term "dependent" only includes a child who has not attained the age of 21 or has not attained the age of 23 and is enrolled in a full-time course of study at an institution of higher learning.

Section 702 of the Ike Skelton National Defense Authorization Act for Fiscal Year 2010 (P.L. 111383)[29] amended title 10, United States Code, to add a new Section 1110b extending coverage to children up to age 26 who are not otherwise eligible to enroll in an employer-sponsored plan to purchase TRICARE coverage. The premium would be equal to the cost of the coverage as determined by the Secretary of Defense on an appropriate actuarial basis. The program is to be effective retroactively, not later than January 1, 2011. On January 13, DOD issued a press release that stated that the program established under this authority will be known as the "TRICARE Young Adult Program."[30] For calendar year 2012 the monthly premium for a TRICARE Young Adult (TYA) Prime enrollment is $201 and $176 for a TYA Standard enrollment.[31]

The premium feature does make the TRICARE program dissimilar from the coverage mandated by ACA. The ACA provision amended the Public Health Service Act to include a Section 2714 that provides:

> A group health plan and a health insurance issuer offering group or individual health insurance coverage that provides dependent coverage of children shall continue to make such coverage available for an adult child (who is not married) until the child turns 26 years of age.

Department of Health and Human Services regulations have interpreted this to extend dependent coverage, not create a new policy for which a separate premium would be charged.[32] Some organizations representing military constituencies have expressed concern about the potential amount of the premiums that might be charged under the new TRICARE program.[33]

Will ACA Extend Coverage to Dependent Children under CHAMPVA up to Age 26?

The provision extending health insurance coverage to dependent children until age 26 in ACA does not appear to extend to CHAMPVA beneficiaries.

In general, eligibility for CHAMPVA is lost when either a child (other than a helpless child)[34] turns 18, unless enrolled in an accredited school as a full-time student; a child, who has been a full-time student, turns 23 or loses full-time student status; a child marries; or a stepchild who no longer lives in the household of the sponsor.

Section 1001 of ACA amends Part A of Title XXVII of the PHSA to add a new Section 2714 specifying that a group health plan and a health insurance issuer offering group or individual health insurance coverage that provides dependent coverage of children shall continue to make such coverage available for an adult child until the child turns 26 years of age. This requirement relating to coverage of adult children will take effect for the plan years beginning on or after September 23, 2010.[35] However, the provisions of Title XXVII of the PHSA do not appear to apply to CHAMPVA.[36] During the 111th Congress, the House-passed version of the National Defense Authorization Act (NDAA) for FY2011 bill (H.R. 5136, H.Rept. 111-491) included a provision that would have extended dependent coverage under CHAMPVA until age 26. However, the final version of the FY2011 NDAA (H.R. 6523; P.L. 111-383) did not include any provision to extend CHAMPVA coverage to eligible dependent children up to age 26.[37] In the 112th Congress, the CHAMPVA Children's Protection Act of 2011 (H.R. 115) has been introduced but has not seen legislative action.

Will ACA Affect the Cost of Prescription Drugs and Medical Devices Provided to Veterans?

It is unclear at this time whether ACA will affect the cost of prescription drugs and medical devices provided to veterans.

Under current law, there are excise taxes on sales by manufacturers of certain products. Certain sales are exempt from this tax.[38] ACA will impose an annual fee on certain manufacturers and importers of branded prescription drugs (including biological products and excluding orphan drugs). The fee structure will be based on annual sales and will be set to reach a certain revenue target each year.[39] In addition, under ACA a new excise tax of 2.3%

will be imposed on the sale of medical devices by manufacturers, producers, or importers.[40] This provision will exempt eyeglasses, contact lenses, hearing aids, and any device of a type that is generally purchased by the public at retail for individual use. The tax will apply to sales made after December 31, 2012.[41]

Section 9011 of ACA requires the Secretary of Veterans Affairs to conduct a study on the effect of provisions in Title IX of ACA—in particular the new fees on drug and device manufacturers—on the cost of medical care provided to veterans, and veterans' access to medical devices and branded prescription drugs. The Secretary is required to report the results of such a study to the House Committee on Ways and Means and the Senate Committee on Finance. The report is required by December 31, 2012.

End Notes

[1] §1501(b) as amended by §10106 (b) of P.L. 111-148 and by §1002 of P.L. 111-152.

[2] §1501 of P.L. 111-148 includes congressional findings that address the constitutionality of an individual mandate to obtain health insurance. For more information on this issue, see CRS Report R40725, *Requiring Individuals to Obtain Health Insurance: A Constitutional Analysis*, by Jennifer Staman et al.

[3] For further details on provisions in PPACA, see CRS Report R41220, *Preexisting Condition Exclusion Provisions for Children and Dependent Coverage under the Patient Protection and Affordable Care Act (ACA)*, by Bernadette Fernandez, Preexisting Exclusion Provisions for Children and Dependent Coverage under the Patient Protection and Affordable Care Act (PPACA), by Hinda Chaikind and Bernadette Fernandez; CRS Report R41166, *Grandfathered Health Plans Under the Patient Protection and Affordable Care Act (PPACA)*, by Bernadette Fernandez; CRS Report R40725, *Requiring Individuals to Obtain Health Insurance: A Constitutional Analysis*, by Jennifer Staman et al.; CRS Report R41586, *Upcoming Rules Pursuant to the Patient Protection and Affordable Care Act: Fall 2010 Unified Agenda*, by Curtis W. Copeland and Maeve P. Carey; CRS Report R41390, *Discretionary Funding in the Patient Protection and Affordable Care Act (ACA)*, coordinated by C. Stephen Redhead; and CRS Report R41128, *Health-Related Revenue Provisions in the Patient Protection and Affordable Care Act (ACA)*, by Janemarie Mulvey.

[4] Michael Posner, "Veterans Push For Fixes To New Law," *Congress Daily*, April 6, 2010.

[5] Jane Norman, "Military Families Left Out of Expanded Health Coverage for Adult Children," *CQ HealthBeat CQ Today*, September 27, 2010.

[6] Ibid. Also see Department of Veterans Affairs, "Statement from VA Secretary Eric K. Shinseki," press release, March 21, 2010, http://www1.va.gov/opa/pressrel/pressrelease. cfm?id=1871; Department of Defense, "Tricare Meets Health Care Bill's Standards, Gates Says," press release, March 22, 2010, http://www.defense.gov//News/NewsArticle. aspx? ID=58412, and Letter from Kathleen Sebelius, Secretary of Health and Human Services, to Honorable Max Baucus, Chairman, Senate Committee on Finance, March 24, 2010, http:// www.tricare.mil/downloads/Baucus%20PPACA.PDF.

[7] For more detailed information on the TRICARE program, see CRS Report RL33537, *Military Medical Care: Questions and Answers*, by Don J. Jansen, and CRS Report RS22402, *Increases in Tricare Costs: Background and Options for Congress*, by Don J. Jansen.

[8] For a complete discussion of eligibility for VA health care, priority groups, and enrollment, see CRS Report R41343, *Veterans Medical Care: FY2011 Appropriations*, by Sidath Viranga Panangala.

[9] U.S. Department of Veterans Affairs, *FY 2008 Performance and Accountability Report*, Washington, DC, November17, 2008, p. 10. Established on January 3, 1946, as the Department of Medicine and Surgery by P.L. 79-293, succeeded in 1989 by the Veterans Health Services and Research Administration, renamed the Veterans Health Administration in 1991.

[10] Adam Oliver, "The Veterans Health Administration: An American Success Story?" *The Milbank Quarterly*, vol. 85, no. 1 (March 2007), pp. 5-35.

[11] Veteran's status is established by active-duty status in the U.S. Armed Forces and an honorable discharge or release from active military service. Generally, persons enlisting in one of the armed forces after September 7, 1980, and officers commissioned after October 16, 1981, must have completed two years of active duty or the full period of their initial service obligation to be eligible for VA health care benefits. Service members discharged at any time because of service-connected disabilities are not held to this requirement.

[12] A service-connected disability is a disability that was incurred or aggravated in the line of duty in the U.S. Armed Forces (38 U.S.C. §101 (16). VA determines whether veterans have service-connected disabilities, and for those with such disabilities, assigns ratings from 0% to 100% based on the severity of the disability. Percentages are assigned in increments of 10% (38 C.F.R. §§4.1-4.31).

[13] For example, veterans who may have been exposed to Agent Orange during the Vietnam War or veterans who may have diseases potentially related to service in the Gulf War may be eligible to receive care.

[14] Veterans with no service-connected conditions and who are Medicaid eligible, or who have an income below a certain VA means-test threshold and below a median income threshold for the geographic area in which they live, are also eligible to enroll in the VA health care system.

[15] A detail listing of VHA's standardized medical benefits package is available at 38 C.F.R. §17.38 (2010).

[16] 38 U.S.C. §1729.

[17] 38 U.S.C. §1729(a)(2)(D); 38 C.F.R. §17.101(a)(1)(i) (2010).

[18] For more information, see CRS Report RS22483, *Health Care for Dependents and Survivors of Veterans*, by Sidath Viranga Panangala.

[19] Veterans Health Care Expansion Act of 1973 (P.L. 93-82).

[20] 38 U.S.C. §1781; 38 C.F.R. §17.270-17.278.

[21] §3110 of PPACA.

[22] 10 U.S.C. §1086(d).

[23] §201, P.L. 111-309.

[24] U.S. Government Accountability Office, *Impact of Health Care Reform Legislation on the Department of Defense*, GAO-11-837R, September 26, 2011, p. 2, http://www.gao.gov/new.items/d11837r.pdf.

[25] See 42 U.S.C. 300gg-91(d)(8).

[26] 38 U.S.C. §§1803; 1821.

[27] 38 U.S.C. §§1811; 1812; 1813.

[28] See 42 U.S.C. §300gg-21(b), as amended by PPACA (containing limitations on the applicability of the Public Health Services Act provisions).

[29] H.R. 6523 signed into law on January 7, 2011.

[30] http://www.tricare.mil/mediacenter/news.aspx?fid=685.

[31] Please see: http://www.tricare.mil/mybenefit/Download/Forms/TRICARE_Summary_of_Beneficiary_Costs_Brochure_2011_LoRes.pdf.

[32] http://www.hhs.gov/ociio/regulations/dependent/index.html.

[33] See for example: http://www.moaa.org/lac_issues_update_101015.htm#issue3.

[34] A helpless child is established after a fact-based analysis completed by a VA Regional Office determines the child to be permanently incapable of self-support by the age of 18. See 38 C.F.R. §3.356 and http://www.va.gov/hac/forbeneficiaries/champva/handbook/chandbook. pdf.

[35] Department of The Treasury, Department of Labor ,and Department of Health and Human Services, "Interim Final Rules for Group Health Plans and Health Insurance Issuers Relating to Dependent Coverage of Children to Age 26 Under the Patient Protection and Affordable Care Act," 75 *Federal Register* 27122-27140, May 12, 2010.

[36] See 42 U.S.C. 300gg-91(b)(1).

[37] During the 111th Congress four stand-alone measures were introduced to extend CHAMPVA coverage to eligible dependent children up to age 26: H.R. 5185, H.R. 5206, S. 3356, and S. 3801.

[38] See Internal Revenue Code Chapter 32.

[39] CRS Report R40943, *Public Health, Workforce, Quality, and Related Provisions in the Patient Protection and Affordable Care Act (P.L. 111-148)*, coordinated by C. Stephen Redhead and Erin D. Williams.

[40] Ibid.

[41] CRS Report R41128, *Health-Related Revenue Provisions in the Patient Protection and Affordable Care Act (ACA)*, by Janemarie Mulvey.

In: Military Health Care
Editor: Brian M. Gagliardi

ISBN: 978-1-62417-339-4
© 2013 Nova Science Publishers, Inc.

Chapter 3

DEFENSE HEALTH CARE: DOD LACKS ASSURANCE THAT SELECTED RESERVE MEMBERS ARE INFORMED ABOUT TRICARE RESERVE SELECT*

United States Government Accountability Office

ABBREVIATIONS

DMDC	Defense Manpower Data Center
DOD	Department of Defense
FEHB	Federal Employees Health Benefits
NDAA	National Defense Authorization Act
TAMP	Transitional Assistance Management Program
TMA	TRICARE Management Activity
TRS	TRICARE Reserve Select

---

* This is an edited, reformatted and augmented version of The United States Government Accountability Office publication, Report to Congressional Committees GAO-11-551, dated June 2011.

WHY GAO DID THIS STUDY

TRICARE Reserve Select (TRS) provides certain members of the Selected Reserve—reservists considered essential to wartime missions—with the ability to purchase health care coverage under the Department of Defense's (DOD) TRICARE program after their active duty coverage expires. TRS is similar to TRICARE Standard, a fee-forservice option, and TRICARE Extra, a preferred provider option.

The National Defense Authorization Act for Fiscal Year 2008 directed GAO to review TRS education and access to care for TRS beneficiaries. This report examines (1) how DOD ensures that members of the Selected Reserve are informed about TRS and (2) how DOD monitors and evaluates access to civilian providers for TRS beneficiaries. GAO reviewed and analyzed documents and evaluated an analysis of claims conducted by DOD. GAO also interviewed officials with the TRICARE Management Activity (TMA), the DOD entity responsible for managing TRICARE; the regional TRICARE contractors; the Office of Reserve Affairs; and the seven reserve components.

WHAT GAO RECOMMENDS

GAO recommends that the Secretary of Defense direct the Assistant Secretary of Defense for Reserve Affairs to develop a policy requiring each reserve component to designate a centralized point of contact for TRS education. DOD partially concurred with this recommendation, citing a concern about regional coordination. GAO modified the recommendation.

WHAT GAO FOUND

DOD does not have reasonable assurance that Selected Reserve members are informed about TRS. A 2007 policy designated the reserve components as having responsibility for providing information about TRS to Selected Reserve members on an annual basis; however, officials from three of the seven components told GAO that they were unaware of this policy. Additionally, only one of the reserve components had a designated official at the headquarters level acting as a central point of contact for TRICARE education, including TRS. Without centralized responsibility for TRS education, the reserve components cannot ensure that all eligible Selected Reserve members are receiving information about the TRS program. Compounding this, the managed care support contractors that manage civilian health care are limited in their ability to educate all reserve component units in their regions as required by their contracts because they do not have access to comprehensive information about these units, and some units choose not to use the contractors to help educate their members about TRS. Nonetheless, DOD officials stated that they were satisfied with the contractors' efforts to educate units upon request and to conduct outreach. Lastly, it is difficult to determine whether Selected Reserve members are knowledgeable about TRS because the results of two DOD surveys that gauged members' awareness of the program may not be representative because of low response rates.

Because TRS is the same benefit as the TRICARE Standard and Extra options, DOD monitors access to civilian providers for TRS beneficiaries in conjunction with TRICARE Standard and Extra beneficiaries. DOD has mainly used feedback mechanisms, such as surveys, to gauge access to civilian providers for these beneficiaries in the absence of access standards for these options. GAO found that jointly monitoring access for these two beneficiary groups is reasonable because a claims analysis showed that TRS beneficiaries and TRICARE Standard and Extra beneficiaries had similar health care utilization. Also, during the course of GAO's review, TMA initiated other efforts that specifically evaluated access to civilian providers for the Selected Reserve population and TRS beneficiaries, including mapping the locations of Selected Reserve members in relation to areas with TRICARE provider networks.

June 3, 2011

The Honorable Carl Levin
Chairman

The Honorable John McCain
Ranking Member
Committee on Armed Services
United States Senate

The Honorable Howard P. "Buck" McKeon
Chairman

The Honorable Adam Smith
Ranking Member
Committee on Armed Services
House of Representatives

Since the September 11, 2001, terrorist attacks, the Department of
Defense (DOD) has increasingly relied on reservists to support military
operations, such as the conflicts in Iraq and Afghanistan. This has increased
both the number of Selected Reserve members—reservists who are considered
essential to wartime missions—supporting DOD's current operations and the
duration of their active duty service.[1] In recognition of this, Congress has
increased the health care benefits available to reservists and their dependents,
which include spouses and dependent children. Specifically, the National
Defense Authorization Acts (NDAA) for Fiscal Years 2004, 2005, 2006, 2007,
and 2010 expanded the number of reservists (including Selected Reserve
members) who qualify for TRICARE, the military health care program, and
increased the period of time during which they qualify.[2] The NDAA for Fiscal
Year 2005 also established the program that DOD has named TRICARE
Reserve Select (TRS), under which most members of the Selected Reserve
who are not on active duty may purchase TRICARE coverage after the
coverage associated with active duty expires. TRS is the same benefit as
TRICARE Standard, a fee-for-service option, and TRICARE Extra, a
preferred provider option. All three programs cover health care provided at
military treatment facilities and through civilian providers, both network
(TRICARE Extra) and nonnetwork (TRICARE Standard).[3] However, unlike
TRICARE beneficiaries who use the Standard and Extra options, TRS
enrollees must pay a monthly premium to receive benefits through the
program.

In recent years, members of Congress have raised questions about whether
reservists, including members of the Selected Reserve, and their dependents
have adequate health insurance when they are not on active duty and whether
they have difficulty using TRICARE when they are eligible for it. In 2007, we
reported on several issues related to reservists, including DOD's efforts to
educate reservists and their dependents about TRICARE benefits, reservists'
satisfaction with TRICARE, and the types of problems that reservists and their
dependents experienced when using TRICARE.[4] We found that DOD was
challenged by the task of educating reservists and their dependents about
TRICARE, and we recommended that DOD provide additional briefings to
reservists and their dependents at specific points in time. We also found that

although a majority of reservists reported that they were satisfied with their TRICARE benefits, some reservists reported experiencing difficulties when using the program, including difficulties understanding TRICARE and difficulties finding a health care provider who accepted TRICARE beneficiaries as patients.

Subsequent to our report, the Commission on the National Guard and Reserves reported to Congress in 2008 that the TRICARE Management Activity (TMA)—the DOD entity responsible for overseeing TRICARE— and the military services have not undertaken a sufficiently aggressive educational campaign to help improve reservists' and their families' understanding of TRICARE.[5] More recently, groups representing military beneficiaries told us that they were concerned about low enrollment within the TRS program, and they questioned whether these enrollment numbers are the result of inadequate education by DOD. According to DOD officials, as of December 2010 about 392,000 of the more than 858,000 members of the Selected Reserve were eligible for TRS.[6] Of these, about 67,000 members (17 percent) had purchased TRS.

Concerns have also been expressed about the ability of reservists, including members of the Selected Reserve, and their families to access health care. In June 2007, DOD's Task Force on Mental Health reported that because reservists may not live near military installations like their active duty counterparts, they may not have convenient access to military hospitals and clinics and must instead rely more heavily on civilian providers for their care.[7]

The NDAA for Fiscal Year 2008 directed us to review DOD's efforts to educate members of the Selected Reserve about TRS and access to care for TRS beneficiaries.[8] This report examines (1) how DOD ensures that members of the Selected Reserve are informed about TRS and (2) how DOD monitors and evaluates access to civilian providers for TRS beneficiaries.

To examine how DOD ensures that members of the Selected Reserve are informed about TRS and how DOD monitors and evaluates access to civilian providers for TRS beneficiaries, we interviewed officials with TMA, including officials with the Warrior Support Branch, which oversees TRS, and officials with the Communications and Customer Service Division, which develops educational materials for TRICARE. We also interviewed officials from each of the three TRICARE Regional Offices (North, South, and West) and officials from each of the regional managed care support contractors (contractors) to discuss their responsibilities for educating members of the Selected Reserve about TRICARE, including TRS, and for ensuring beneficiaries' access to civilian providers. In addition, we interviewed officials from military coalition groups that represent reservists to obtain their perspectives on TRS education and access to civilian providers. To identify TRS education requirements, we reviewed and analyzed policy guidelines and TRICARE managed care support contract requirements. We interviewed officials with the Office of Reserve Affairs as well as officials from each of the seven reserve components to identify their role in educating the Selected Reserve about TRICARE. We also reviewed relevant standards for internal control in the federal government.[9] Additionally, we evaluated two surveys conducted by DOD that collected information on whether members of the Selected Reserve were aware of the TRS program—the Status of Forces Survey and the *Focused Survey of TRICARE Reserve Select and Selected Reserve Military Health System Access and Satisfaction.*

To determine how DOD monitors and evaluates access to civilian providers for TRS, we reviewed TMA's beneficiary surveys on access to civilian providers under TRICARE Standard, TRICARE Extra, and TRS. We also reviewed the TRICARE Regional Offices' recent efforts to evaluate the adequacy of access to civilian providers under the TRICARE Standard, TRICARE Extra, and TRS options. Additionally, we evaluated an analysis of claims conducted by TMA—at our request—that compared claims filed by TRICARE Standard and Extra beneficiaries with those filed by TRS beneficiaries for fiscal years 2008 through 2010 to identify demographic differences between these populations and to determine whether these populations used similar types of providers and obtained similar types of care. We assessed the reliability of these data by speaking with knowledgeable officials and reviewing related documentation, and we determined that the claims analyses presented in this report are sufficiently reliable for our purposes. (See app. I for more detail about the claims analyses.) We also reviewed efforts by TMA to identify locations of the Selected Reserve members and analyze whether they resided within an area that was served by a TRICARE provider network. Finally, we reviewed TMA's efforts to repeat its survey that is specific to the TRS program (Focused Survey of TRICARE Reserve Select and Selected Reserve Military Health System Access and Satisfaction).

We conducted this performance audit from July 2010 through June 2011 in accordance with generally accepted government auditing standards. Those standards require that we plan and perform the audit to obtain sufficient, appropriate evidence to provide a reasonable basis for our findings and conclusions based on our audit objectives. We believe that the evidence obtained provides a reasonable basis for our findings and conclusions based on our audit objectives.

BACKGROUND

Reservists are members of the seven reserve components, which provide trained and qualified persons available for active duty in the armed forces in time of war or national emergency.

The Selected Reserve is the largest category of reservists and is designated as essential to wartime missions.[10] The Selected Reserve is also the only category of reservists that is eligible for TRS. As of December 31, 2010, the Selected Reserve included 858,997 members dispersed among the seven reserve components with about two-thirds belonging to the Army Reserve and the Army National Guard.[11]

See figure 1 for the number and percentage of Selected Reserve members within each reserve component.

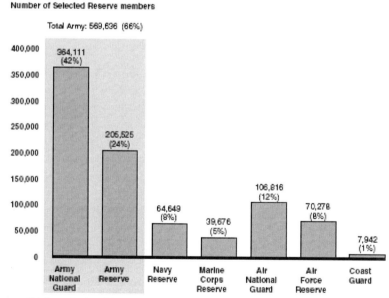

Source: GAO analysis of Department of Defense data.

Figure 1. Number of Selected Reserve Members by Component as a Percentage of All Selected Reserve Members, December 31, 2010.

Additionally, about two-thirds of the Selected Reserve members are 35 years old or younger (64 percent) and about half are single (52 percent). (See fig. 2.)

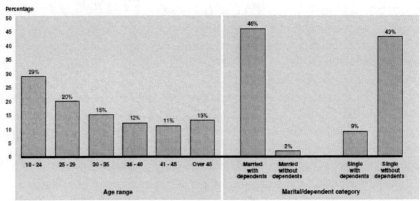

Source: GAO analysis of Department of Defense data.

Figure 2. Age and Marital Status of Selected Reserve Members, December 31, 2010.

History of TRS

The NDAA for Fiscal Year 2005 authorized the TRS program and made TRICARE coverage available to certain members of the Selected Reserve.[12] The program was subsequently expanded and restructured by the NDAAs for Fiscal Years 2006 and 2007[13]—although additional program changes were made in subsequent years.[14]

- In fiscal year 2005, to qualify for TRS, members of the Selected Reserve had to enter into an agreement with their respective reserve components to continue to serve in the Selected Reserve in exchange for TRS coverage, and they were given 1 year of TRS eligibility for every 90 days served in support of a contingency operation.[15]
- The NDAA for Fiscal Year 2006, which became effective on October 1, 2006, expanded the program, and almost all members of the Selected Reserve and their dependents—regardless of their prior active duty service—had the option of purchasing TRICARE coverage through a monthly premium. The portion of the premium paid by the members of the Selected Reserve and their dependents for

TRS coverage varied based on certain qualifying conditions that had to be met, such as whether the member of the Selected Reserve also had access to an employer-sponsored health plan. The NDAA for Fiscal Year 2006 established two levels—which DOD called tiers—of qualification for TRS, in addition to the tier established by the NDAA for Fiscal Year 2005, with enrollees paying different portions of the premium based on the tier for which they qualified.[16]

- The NDAA for Fiscal Year 2007 significantly restructured the TRS program by eliminating the three-tiered premium structure and establishing open enrollment for members of the Selected Reserve provided that they are not eligible for or currently enrolled in the FEHB Program.17 The act removed the requirement that members of the Selected Reserve sign service agreements to qualify for TRS. Instead, the act established that members of the Selected Reserve qualify for TRS for the duration of their service in the Selected Reserve. DOD implemented these changes on October 1, 2007.

TRICARE Options and Cycle of Coverage for the Selected Reserve

Generally, TRICARE provides its benefits through several options for its non-Medicare-eligible beneficiary population.[18] These options vary according to TRICARE beneficiary enrollment requirements, the choices TRICARE beneficiaries have in selecting civilian and military treatment facility providers, and the amount TRICARE beneficiaries must contribute toward the cost of their care. Table 1 provides information about these options.

Selected Reserve members have a cycle of coverage during which they are eligible for different TRICARE options based on their duty status—preactivation, active duty, deactivation, and inactive. During preactivation, when members of the Selected Reserve are notified that they will serve on active duty in support of a contingency operation in the near future, they and their families are eligible to enroll in TRICARE Prime, and therefore, they do not need to purchase TRS coverage.[19] This is commonly referred to as "early eligibility" and continues uninterrupted once members of the Selected Reserve begin active duty. While on active duty, members are required to enroll in TRICARE Prime. Similarly during deactivation, for 180 days after returning from active duty in support of a contingency operation, members of the Selected Reserve are rendered eligible for the Transitional Assistance

Management Program, a program to transition back to civilian life in which members and dependents can use the TRICARE Standard or Extra options.[20] When members of the Selected Reserve return to inactive status, they can choose to purchase TRS coverage if eligible.

Table 1. Summary of TRICARE Options

TRICARE option	Description
TRICARE Prime	Active duty servicemembers are required to enroll in this managed care option while other TRICARE beneficiaries may choose to enroll in this option. TRICARE Prime enrollees receive most of their care from providers at military treatment facilities, augmented by network civilian providers. TRICARE Prime offers lower out-of-pocket costs than the other TRICARE options. It is also the only option with access standards, which include appointment wait times and travel times.
TRICARE Standard and TRICARE Extra	TRICARE beneficiaries, who are not on active duty, who choose not to enroll in TRICARE Prime may obtain health care from nonnetwork civilian providers (under TRICARE Standard) or network civilian providers (under TRICARE Extra). Under TRICARE Extra, beneficiaries have lower cost-shares than they would have under the TRICARE Standard option—about 5 percentage points less for using network providers.
TRICARE Reserve Select (TRS)	TRS is a premium-based health plan that certain members of the Selected Reserve, who are not on active duty, may purchase. Under TRS, beneficiaries may obtain health care from either nonnetwork or network civilian providers, similar to beneficiaries using TRICARE Standard or Extra, respectively, and will pay lower cost-shares for using network providers.

Source: GAO summary of Department of Defense TRICARE documentation.
Note: All beneficiaries may obtain care at military treatment facilities although priority is first given to active duty personnel and then TRICARE Prime enrollees.

As a result of the TRICARE coverage cycle and program eligibility requirements, TMA officials estimate that at any given time, fewer than half of the members of the Selected Reserve are qualified to purchase TRS. Currently, to qualify for TRS, a member of the Selected Reserve must not

- be eligible for the FEHB Program,
- have been notified that he or she will serve on active duty in support of a contingency operation, and

- be serving on active duty or have recently, that is, within 180 days, returned from active duty in support of a contingency operation.

Of the more than 390,000 members eligible, about 67,000 members were enrolled in TRS as of December 31, 2010. (See fig. 3.)

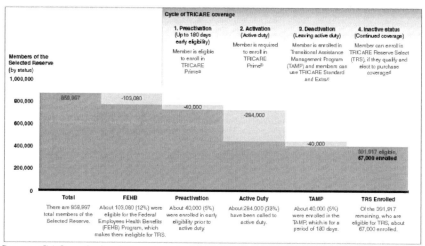

Source: GAO analysis of Department of Defense data.

[a] If a Selected Reserve member was enrolled in TRS prior to preactivation, the member is automatically disenrolled at this time. Even if a member does not enroll, the member will receive TRICARE benefits. In addition, at this time, members and their families begin receiving the same care as active duty servicemembers and their families. This is applicable when a member of the Selected Reserve is called to active duty for more than 30 days and is serving in support of a contingency operation.

[b] Even if a member does not enroll he or she will still receive TRICARE Prime benefits.

[c] TAMP is applicable when a member of the Selected Reserve is called to active duty for more than 30 days and is serving in support of a contingency operation. TRICARE Prime is available in specific locations.

[d] If a member was enrolled in TRS prior to serving on active duty, the member must reenroll after returning to inactive status. Members are not automatically reenrolled in TRS; they must requalify and purchase TRS again. In addition, the cycle repeats once a Selected Reserve member is called to active duty.

Figure 3. Cycle of TRICARE Coverage and Eligibility as of December 31, 2010.

DOD Entities Involved with TRS

A number of different DOD entities have various responsibilities related to TRS.

- Within the Office of the Under Secretary of Defense for Personnel and Readiness, the Office of the Assistant Secretary of Defense for Reserve Affairs works with the seven reserve components to determine whether members of the Selected Reserve are eligible for TRS and to ensure that members have information about TRICARE, including TRS.
- Within TMA, the Warrior Support Branch is responsible for managing the TRS option, which includes developing policy and regulations. This office also works with TMA's Communication and Customer Service Division to develop educational materials for this program. The Assistant Secretary of Defense for Health Affairs oversees TMA and reports to the Under Secretary of Defense for Personnel and Readiness.
- TMA works with contractors to manage civilian health care and other services in each TRICARE region (North, South, and West).21 The contractors are required to establish and maintain sufficient networks of civilian providers within certain designated areas, called Prime Service Areas, to ensure access to civilian providers for all TRICARE beneficiaries, regardless of enrollment status or Medicare eligibility.22 They are also responsible for helping TRICARE beneficiaries locate providers and for informing and educating TRICARE beneficiaries and providers on all aspects of the TRICARE program, including TRS.
- TMA's TRICARE Regional Offices, located in each of the three TRICARE regions, are responsible for managing health care delivery for all TRICARE options in their respective geographic areas and overseeing the contractors, including monitoring network quality and adequacy, monitoring customer satisfaction outcomes, and coordinating appointment and referral management policies.

DOD DOES NOT HAVE REASONABLE ASSURANCE THAT SELECTED RESERVE MEMBERS ARE INFORMED ABOUT TRS

DOD does not have reasonable assurance that members of the Selected Reserve are informed about TRS for several reasons. First, the reserve components do not have a centralized point of contact to ensure that members are educated about the program. Second, the contractors are challenged in their ability to educate the reserve component units in their respective regions because they do not have comprehensive information about the units in their areas of responsibility. And, finally, DOD cannot say with certainty whether Selected Reserve members are knowledgeable about TRS because the results of two surveys that gauged members' awareness of the program may not be representative of the Selected Reserve population because of low response rates.

Reserve Components Are Responsible for Providing Information about TRS to Selected Reserve Members, but Most Components Have Not Established Centralized Accountability for TRS Education

A 2007 policy from the Under Secretary of Defense for Personnel and Readiness designated the reserve components as having responsibility for providing information about TRS to members of the Selected Reserve at least once a year. When the policy was first issued, officials from the Office of Reserve Affairs—who have oversight responsibility for the reserve components—told us that they met with officials from each of the reserve components to discuss how the components would fulfill this responsibility. However, according to officials from the Office of Reserve Affairs, they have not met with the reserve components since 2008 to discuss how the components are fulfilling their TRS education responsibilities under the policy. These officials explained that they have experienced difficulties identifying a representative from each of the reserve components to attend meetings about TRS education. When we contacted officials from all seven reserve components to discuss TRS education, we had similar experiences. Three of the components had difficulties providing a point of contact. In fact, two of the components took several months to identify an official whom we could speak with about TRS education, and the other one had difficulties identifying someone who could answer our follow-up questions when our original point of contact was no longer available. Furthermore, officials from three of the seven components told us that they were not aware of this policy.

Regardless of their knowledge of the 2007 policy, officials from all of the reserve components told us that education responsibilities are delegated to their unit commanders. These responsibilities include informing members about their health options, which would include TRS. All of the components provide various means of support to their unit commanders to help fulfill this responsibility.[23] For example, three of the components provide information about TRICARE directly to their unit commanders or the commanders' designees through briefings. The four other components provide information to their unit commanders through other means, such as policy documents, Web sites, and newsletters.

Additionally, while most of the components had someone designated to answer TRICARE benefit questions, only one of the reserve components had an official at the headquarters level designated as a central point of contact for TRICARE education, including TRS.[24] This official told us that he was unaware of the specific 2007 TRS education policy; however, he said his responsibilities for TRS education include developing annual communication plans, providing briefings to unit commanders, and publishing articles in the Air Force magazine about TRS. Designating a point of contact is important because a key factor in meeting standards for internal control in federal agencies is defining and assigning key areas of authority and responsibility— such as a point of contact for a specific policy. Without a point of contact to ensure that this policy is implemented, the reserve components are running the risk that some of their Selected Reserve members may not be receiving information about the TRS program—especially since some of the reserve component officials we met with were unaware of the policy.

TRICARE Contractors Are Challenged in Their Ability to Annually Brief Reserve Component Units about TRS Because They Lack Comprehensive Information about the Units

The TRICARE contractors are required to provide an annual briefing about TRS to each reserve component unit in their regions, including both Reserve and National Guard units. All three contractors told us that they maintain education representatives who are responsible for educating members of the Selected Reserve on TRS. These representatives conduct unit outreach and provide information to members of the Selected Reserve at any time during predeployment and demobilization, at family events, and during drill weekends. The contractors use briefing materials maintained by TMA and posted on the TRICARE Web site. In addition to conducting briefings, the three contractors have increased their outreach efforts in various ways, including creating an online tutorial that explains TRS, mailing TRS information to Selected Reserve members, and working closely with Family Program coordinators to provide TRS information to family members.

However, the contractors are challenged in their ability to meet their requirement for briefing all units annually. First, they typically provide briefings to units upon request because this approach is practical based upon units' schedules and availability. For example, officials from one contractor told us that even though they know when geographically dispersed units will be gathering in one location, these units have busy schedules and may not have time for the contractor to provide a briefing. Each contractor records the briefings that are requested, when the briefing requests were fulfilled and by whom, and any questions or concerns that resulted from the briefings. However, some unit commanders do not request briefings from the contractors. For example, officials with one reserve component told us that they do not rely on the contractor to brief units because they were unaware that the contractors provided this service. In addition, these officials as well as officials from another reserve component told us that they did not know if their unit commanders were aware that they could request briefings from the contractors. All of the contractors told us that they conduct outreach to offer information to some of the units that have not requested a briefing, including both calling units to offer a briefing and providing materials. They added that more outreach is conducted to National Guard units because they are able to obtain information about these units from state officials. The TRICARE Regional Offices also told us that they conduct outreach to units to let them know that the contractor is available to brief the units about TRS. However, even though the contractor and the TRICARE Regional Offices conduct outreach to a unit, it does not necessarily mean that the unit will request a briefing.

Furthermore, while contractors are aware of some units in their regions, they do not have access to comprehensive lists of all reserve component units in their regions because the Web site links containing unit information that TMA originally provided to the contractors have become inactive. As a result, the contractors are not able to verify whether all units in their regions have received briefings. Officials from the Office of Reserve Affairs told us that reserve components report unit information to the Defense Manpower Data

Center (DMDC), which maintains personnel information about all members of the military.

However, these officials raised concerns about the accuracy of this information because it could be about 3 to 6 months old and may not be comprehensive. Officials at the Office of Reserve Affairs told us that the reserve components would likely have more up-to-date information about their units as they are responsible for reporting this information to DMDC. However, officials from TMA, the TRICARE Regional Offices, and contractors also told us that a comprehensive list of units would be difficult to maintain because the unit structure changes frequently.

Despite the challenges contractors face, officials with TMA's Warrior Support Branch told us that they are satisfied with the contractors' efforts to provide TRS briefings to the reserve component units in their regions. However, because officials do not know which units have been briefed on the program, there is a risk that some reserve component members are not receiving sufficient information on TRS and may not be taking advantage of coverage available to them.

DOD has conducted two surveys that gauge whether members of the Selected Reserve are aware of TRS, among other issues. In 2008, TMA conducted the *Focused Survey of TRICARE Reserve Select and Selected Reserve Military Health System Access and Satisfaction* to better understand reserve component members' motivation for enrolling in TRS and to compare TRS enrollees' satisfaction with and access to health care services with that of other beneficiary groups.[25] In reporting the results of this survey to Congress in February 2009, TMA stated that lack of awareness was an important factor in why eligible members of the Selected Reserve did not enroll in TRS.[26] TMA also reported that less than half of the eligible Selected Reserve members who were not enrolled in TRS were aware of the program.[27] However, the survey's response rate was almost 18 percent, and such a low response rate decreases the likelihood that the survey results were representative of the views and characteristics of the Selected Reserve population.

According to the Office of Management and Budget's standards for statistical surveys, a nonresponse analysis is recommended for surveys with response rates lower than 80 percent to determine whether the responses are representative of the surveyed population.

Accordingly, TMA conducted a nonresponse analysis to determine whether the survey responses it received were representative of the surveyed population, and the analysis identified substantial differences between the original respondents and the follow-up respondents. As a result of the differences found in the nonresponse analysis, TMA adjusted the statistical weighting techniques for nonresponse bias and applied the weights to the data before drawing conclusions and reporting the results.

DMDC conducts a quarterly survey, called the Status of Forces Survey, which is directed to all members of the military services. DMDC conducts several versions of this survey, including a version for members of the reserve components.

This survey focuses on different issues at different points in time. For example, every other year the survey includes questions on health benefits, including questions on whether members of the reserve components are aware of TRICARE, including TRS.

In July 2010, we issued a report raising concerns about the reliability of DOD's Status of Forces Surveys because they generally have a 25 to 42 percent response rate, and DMDC has not been conducting nonresponse analyses to determine whether the surveys' results are representative of the target population.[28]

We recommended that DMDC develop and implement guidance both for conducting a nonresponse analysis and using the results of this analysis to inform DMDC's statistical weighting techniques, as part of the collection and analysis of the Status of Forces Survey results.

DOD concurred with this recommendation, but as of January 2011, had not implemented it.

DOD MONITORS ACCESS TO CIVILIAN PROVIDERS UNDER TRS IN CONJUNCTION WITH OTHER TRICARE OPTIONS AND HAS TAKEN STEPS TO EVALUATE ACCESS SPECIFICALLY FOR TRS

DOD monitors access to civilian providers under TRS in conjunction with monitoring efforts related to the TRICARE Standard and Extra options. In addition, during the course of our review, TMA initiated additional efforts that specifically examine access to civilian providers for TRS beneficiaries and the Selected Reserve population, including mapping the locations of Selected Reserve members in relation to areas with TRICARE provider networks.

DOD Monitors Access to Civilian Providers for TRS Beneficiaries along with TRICARE Standard and Extra Beneficiaries

Because TRS is the same benefit as the TRICARE Standard and Extra options, DOD monitors TRS beneficiaries' access to civilian providers as a part of monitoring access to civilian providers for beneficiaries who use TRICARE Standard and Extra.

As we have recently reported, in the absence of access-to-care standards for these options, TMA has mainly used feedback mechanisms to gauge access to civilian providers for these beneficiaries.[29]

For example, in response to a mandate included in the NDAA for Fiscal Year 2008, DOD has completed 2 years of a multiyear survey of beneficiaries who use the TRICARE Standard, TRICARE Extra, and TRS options and 2 years of its second multiyear survey of civilian providers. Congress required that these surveys obtain information on access to care and that DOD give a high priority to locations having high concentrations of Selected Reserve members.

In March 2010, we reported that TMA generally addressed the methodological requirements outlined in the mandate during the implementation of the first year of the multiyear surveys.[30] While TMA did not give a high priority to locations with high concentrations of Selected Reserve members, TMA's methodological approach over the 4-year survey period will cover the entire United States, including areas with high concentrations of Selected Reserve members.

In February 2010, TMA directed the TRICARE Regional Offices to monitor access to civilian providers for TRICARE Standard, TRICARE Extra, and TRS beneficiaries through the development of a model that can be used to identify geographic areas where beneficiaries may experience access problems.

As of May 2010, each of the TRICARE Regional Offices had implemented an initial model appropriate to its region. These models include, for example, data on area populations, provider types, and potential provider shortages for the general population.

Officials at each regional office said that their models are useful but noted that they are evolving and will be updated.

To determine whether jointly monitoring access to civilian providers for TRS beneficiaries along with TRICARE Standard and Extra beneficiaries was reasonable, we asked TMA to perform an analysis of claims (for fiscal years

2008, 2009, and 2010) to identify differences in age demographics and health care utilization between these beneficiary groups.

This analysis found that although the age demographics for these populations were different—more than half of the TRS beneficiaries were age 29 and under, while more than half of the TRICARE Standard and Extra beneficiaries were over 45—both groups otherwise shared similarities with their health care utilization.[31] Specifically, both beneficiary groups had similar diagnoses, used the same types of specialty providers, and used similar proportions of mental health care, primary care, and specialty care. (See fig. 4.) Specifically:

- Seven of the top 10 diagnoses for both TRS and TRICARE Standard and Extra beneficiaries were the same. Three of these diagnoses—allergic rhinitis,[32] joint disorder, and back disorder—made up more than 20 percent of claims for both beneficiary groups.
- The five provider specialties that filed the most claims for both beneficiary groups were the same—family practice, physical therapy, allergy, internal medicine, and pediatrics. Furthermore, the majority of claims filed for both beneficiary groups were filed by family practice providers.
- Both beneficiary groups had the same percentage of claims filed for mental health care and similar percentages for primary care and other specialty care. (See app. II for additional details on the results of this claims analysis.)

Based on this analysis, jointly monitoring access for TRS beneficiaries and TRICARE Standard and Extra beneficiaries appears to be a reasonable approach.

DOD Has Taken Steps to Separately Evaluate Access to Civilian Providers for the Selected Reserve Population and TRS Beneficiaries

DOD has taken steps to evaluate access to civilian providers for the Selected Reserve population and TRS beneficiaries separately from other TRICARE beneficiaries.

Specifically, during the course of our review, TMA initiated the following efforts:

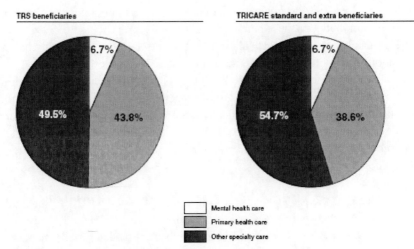

Source: GAO analysis of TRICARE Management Activity data.

Figure 4. Proportion of Claims Filed by TRICARE Reserve Select and TRICARE Standard and Extra Beneficiaries for Mental Health, Primary, and Other Specialty Care, Fiscal Years 2008 through 2010.

- During the fall of 2010, TMA officials analyzed the locations of Selected Reserve members and their families, including TRS beneficiaries, to determine what percentage of them live within TRICARE's Prime Service Areas (areas in which the managed care contractors are required to establish and maintain sufficient networks of civilian providers). According to these data, as of August 31, 2010, over 80 percent of Selected Reserve members and their families lived in Prime Service Areas: 100 percent in the South region, which is all Prime Service Areas, and over 70 percent in the North and West regions.[33]
- TMA officials told us that they are repeating the *Focused Survey of TRICARE Reserve Select and Select Reserve Military Health System Access and Satisfaction*, which had first been conducted in 2008. Using results from its first survey, TMA reported to Congress in February 2009 that members of the Selected Reserve who were enrolled in TRS were pleased with access and quality of care under their plan. However, as we have noted, the response rate for this survey was almost 18 percent, although TMA took steps to adjust the data prior to reporting the results. Officials told us that the follow-up survey will focus on whether access to care for TRS beneficiaries has

changed. Officials sent the survey instrument to participants in January 2011. Officials told us that they anticipate results will be available during the summer of 2011.

CONCLUSION

TRS is an important option for members of the Selected Reserve. However, educating this population about TRS has been challenging, and despite efforts by the reserve components and the contractors, some members of the Selected Reserve are likely still unaware of this option. Most of the reserve components lack centralized accountability for TRS education, making it unclear if all members are getting information about the program—a concern that is further exacerbated by the lack of awareness about the TRS education policy among officials from some of the reserve components. Additionally, the contractors' limitations in briefing all of the units in their regions about TRS make each component's need for a central point of contact more evident.

Without centralized accountability, the reserve components do not have assurance that all members of the Selected Reserve who may need TRS have the information they need to take advantage of the health care options available to them.

RECOMMENDATION
FOR EXECUTIVE ACTION

We recommend that the Secretary of Defense direct the Assistant Secretary of Defense for Reserve Affairs to develop a policy that requires each reserve component to designate a centralized point of contact for TRS education, who will be accountable for ensuring that the reserve components are providing information about TRS to their Selected Reserve members annually.

In establishing responsibilities for the centralized points of contact, DOD should explicitly task them with coordinating with their respective TRICARE Regional Offices to ensure that contractors are provided information on the number and location of reserve component units in their regions.

AGENCY COMMENTS AND OUR EVALUATION

In commenting on a draft of this report, DOD partially concurred with our recommendation. Specifically, DOD agreed that the Assistant Secretary of Defense for Reserve Affairs should develop a policy that requires each of the seven reserve components to designate a central point of contact for TRS education that will be accountable for providing information about TRS to their Selected Reserve members annually. However, DOD countered that each designee should coordinate the provision of reserve unit information through the TRICARE Regional Offices rather than communicating directly with the TRICARE contractors, noting that the TRICARE Regional Offices have oversight responsibility for the contractors in their respective regions. We understand the department's concern about coordinating contractor communications through the TRICARE Regional Offices, and we have modified our recommendation accordingly. DOD also provided technical comments, which we incorporated where appropriate.

Randall B. Williamson
Director, Health Care

APPENDIX I: TRICARE MANAGEMENT ACTIVITY ANALYSIS OF CLAIMS

We asked the TRICARE Management Activity (TMA) to conduct an analysis of claims filed for TRICARE Reserve Select (TRS) beneficiaries and TRICARE Standard and Extra beneficiaries. We requested claims data for the most recent three complete fiscal years—2008, 2009, and 2010— based on the fact that the program last experienced changes with eligibility and premiums in fiscal year 2007.1 For the purpose of this analysis, claims consist of all services provided by a professional in an office or other setting outside of an institution.

Records of services rendered at a hospital or other institution were excluded from this analysis. In addition, records for medical supplies and from chiropractors and pharmacies were also excluded. We asked TMA to conduct the following comparative analyses for TRS beneficiaries and TRICARE Standard and Extra beneficiaries:

1. Demographics, including age for each year and averaged over 3 years
2. Percentage of claims filed for primary care, mental health, and other specialists each year for 3 years
3. The top 10 procedures in ranking order made each year and the average over 3 years
4. The top 10 primary diagnoses in ranking order made each year and the average over 3 years
5. The top five provider specialties in ranking order visited each year and the average over 3 years
6. Percentage of claims filed for the top five provider specialties and the average over 3 years

To ensure that TMA's data were sufficiently reliable, we conducted data reliability assessments of the data sets that we used to assess their quality and methodological soundness.

Our review consisted of (1) examining documents that described the respective data, (2) interviewing TMA officials about the data collection and analysis processes, and (3) interviewing TMA officials about internal controls in place to ensure that data are complete and accurate.

We found that all of the data sets used in this report were sufficiently reliable for our purposes. However, we did not independently verify TMA's calculations.

APPENDIX II: CLAIMS FILED FOR TRICARE RESERVE SELECT AND TRICARE STANDARD AND EXTRA BENEFICIARIES

Tables 2 through 5 contain information on claims filed for TRICARE Reserve Select and TRICARE Standard and Extra beneficiaries.

Table 2. Percentage of Claims Filed for TRICARE Reserve Select (TRS) and TRICARE Standard and Extra Beneficiaries by Age of Beneficiary, Fiscal Years 2008 through 2010

Age	Sex	TRICARE Standard and Extra				TRS			
		FY 2008	FY 2009	FY 2010	Total	FY 2008	FY 2009	FY 2010	Total
Under 18	Female	9.3	9.4	9.8	9.5	16.8	16.4	16.0	16.3
	Male	10.0	10.3	10.9	10.4	20.6	20.0	19.8	20.0

Table 2. (Continued)

| Age | Sex | TRICARE Standard and Extra | | | | | TRS | | |
		FY 2008	FY 2009	FY 2010	Total	FY 2008	FY 2009	FY 2010	*Total*
18-24	Female	4.4	4.7	5.0	4.7	6.3	6.7	7.0	*6.8*
	Male	1.8	1.9	2.0	1.9	4.0	4.1	4.5	*4.3*
25-29	Female	1.7	2.0	2.3	2.0	5.9	7.3	7.8	*7.3*
	Male	0.3	0.3	0.4	0.3	4.1	4.9	5.4	*5.0*
30-35	Female	2.2	2.3	2.6	2.4	7.4	7.7	7.8	*7.7*
	Male	0.3	0.3	0.3	0.3	4.0	4.5	4.7	*4.5*
36-40	Female	2.8	2.8	2.8	2.8	6.6	6.1	5.5	*5.9*
	Male	0.4	0.3	0.4	0.4	4.1	3.8	4.2	*4.0*
41-45	Female	4.4	4.1	3.9	4.2	5.4	5.1	4.8	*5.0*
	Male	1.2	1.1	1.0	1.1	3.7	3.2	3.1	*3.2*
Over 45	Female	41.2	40.3	39.0	40.1	6.7	5.9	5.5	*5.9*
	Male	20.2	20.1	19.7	20.0	4.5	4.4	4.0	*4.2*
Total		100.0	100.0	100.0	100.0	100.0	100.0	100.0	*100.0*

Source: GAO analysis of TRICARE Management Activity data.

Table 3. Percentage of Claims Filed for TRICARE Reserve Select (TRS) and TRICARE Standard and Extra Beneficiaries by Mental Health Care, Primary Health Care, and Other Types of Specialty Care, Fiscal Years 2008 through 2010

| | TRICARE Standard and Extra | | | | TRS | | | |
	FY 2008	FY 2009	FY 2010	Total	FY 2008	FY 2009	FY 2010	Total
Mental health care	6.8	6.6	6.7	6.7	7.1	6.6	6.7	6.7
Other specialty care	54.5	54.8	54.8	54.7	49.9	49.4	49.4	49.5
Primary health care	38.7	38.6	38.5	38.6	43.0	44.1	43.9	43.8
Total	100.0	100.0	100.0	100.0	100.0	100.0	100.0	100.0

Source: GAO analysis of TRICARE Management Activity data.

Table 4. Percentage of Claims Filed for TRICARE Reserve Select (TRS) and TRICARE Standard and Extra Beneficiaries by Top 10 Diagnoses in Ranking Order, Fiscal Years 2008 through 2010

| | TRICARE Standard and Extra | | TRS | |
Rank	Diagnoses	Percentage of services	Diagnoses	Percentage of services
1	Allergic rhinitis[a]	12.1	Allergic rhinitis	14.2
2	Joint disorder neck and nose	4.8	Health supervision child[b]	5.5

Rank	TRICARE Standard and Extra		TRS	
	Diagnoses	Percentage of services	Diagnoses	Percentage of services
3	Back disorder neck and nose	3.5	Joint disorder neck and nose	4.5
4	Essential hypertension[c]	2.3	Back disorder neck and nose	3.0
5	Affective psychoses[d]	2.2	Adjustment reaction[e]	2.3
6	Peripheral Enthesopathies[f]	2.1	Special examinations[g]	2.1
7	Health supervision child	2.1	Affective psychoses	1.8
8	Diabetes mellitus[h]	1.7	Asthma[i]	1.8
9	Adjustment reaction	1.7	Acute upper respiratory infections of multiple or unspecified sites	1.6
10	Special examinations	1.7	Suppurative and unspecified otitis media[j]	1.5
	Other diagnoses[k]	65.7	Other diagnoses	61.7

Source: GAO analysis of TRICARE Management Activity data.

[a] Allergic rhinitis is a collection of symptoms, mostly in the nose and eyes, which occur when inhaling an allergen, such as dust, dander, or pollen.

[b] Health supervision of a child refers to the routine medical examination of an infant or child.

[c] Essential hypertension refers to high blood pressure with no identifiable cause.

[d] Affective psychoses is a group of mental disorders, usually recurrent, in which a severe disturbance of mood is accompanied by one or more of the following: delusions, perplexity, disturbed attitude to self, or disorder of perception and behavior.

[e] Adjustment reaction refers to the reaction to chronic stress, including grief and prolonged depression.

[f] Peripheral Enthesopathies refers to a group of disorders of muscles and tendons and their attachments, such as rotator cuff syndrome.

[g] Special examinations refers to routine exams, such as examinations related to vision care, dental care, and pregnancy tests or other gynecological examinations

[h] Diabetes mellitus comprises a group of heterogeneous disorders that have an increase in blood glucose concentrations. The current classifications for diabetes mellitus Types 1 through 4.

[i] Asthma is an inflammatory disorder of the airways, which causes attacks of wheezing, shortness of breath, chest tightness, and coughing.

[j] Suppurative and unspecified otitis media refers to a group of disorders related to the ear, such as the rupturing of the ear drum.

[k] Other diagnoses include any claims filed for medical diagnoses not outlined as top 10 diagnoses above.

Table 5. Percentage of Claims Filed for TRICARE Reserve Select (TRS) and TRICARE Standard and Extra Beneficiaries by Top Five Provider Specialties, Fiscal Years 2008 through 2010

Provider specialty	TRICARE Standard and Extra	TRS
Family practice	15.7	16.0
Physical therapist	11.6	10.8
Allergy	9.8	13.6
Internal medicine	8.9	5.1
Pediatrics	6.8	14.7
Other specialties	47.2	39.9

Source: GAO analysis of TRICARE Management Activity data.

End Notes

[1] For the purposes of this report, the term reservist includes all members of the seven reserve components, which include the Army National Guard, Army Reserve, Navy Reserve, Marine Corps Reserve, Air National Guard, Air Force Reserve, and Coast Guard. There are different categories of reservists within the seven reserve components. The Selected Reserve is the largest category of reservists among the components and has priority over all other categories of reservists.

[2] Prior to these expansions, a reservist and his or her dependents were eligible for TRICARE only while the reservist was serving on active duty for more than 30 days.

[3] Network providers are TRICARE-authorized providers who enter a contractual agreement to provide health care to TRICARE beneficiaries. Nonnetwork providers are TRICARE-authorized providers who do not have a contractual agreement to provide care to TRICARE beneficiaries. All beneficiaries may obtain care at military treatment facilities although priority is first given to any active duty personnel and then to beneficiaries using TRICARE Prime, another TRICARE option, which requires the beneficiary to enroll.

[4] GAO, Military Health: Increased TRICARE Eligibility for Reservists Presents Educational Challenges, GAO-07-195 (Washington, D.C.: Feb. 12, 2007).

[5] Commission on the National Guard and Reserves, Transforming the National Guard and Reserves into a 21st-Century Operational Force: Final Report to Congress and the Secretary of Defense (Washington D.C., 2008).

[6] To qualify for TRS, a member of the Selected Reserve of a reserve component must not be eligible for or enrolled in the Federal Employees Health Benefits (FEHB) Program either under his or her own eligibility or through a family member. See 10 U.S.C. § 1076d. All National Guard and Reserve manpower is assigned to one of three reserve component categories—the Ready Reserve, the Standby Reserve, and the Retired Reserve. 10 U.S.C. § 10141(a). The Selected Reserve is a component of the Ready Reserve. Once activated to duty, National Guard and Reserve servicemembers are eligible for TRICARE Prime.

[7] Department of Defense, Task Force on Mental Health, An Achievable Vision: Report of the Department of Defense Task Force on Mental Health (Falls Church, Va., June 2007).

[8] Pub. L. No. 110-181, § 711(b)(2)(G), (H), 122 Stat. 3, 192 (2008).

[9] Standards for internal control in the federal government state that agency management is responsible for establishing and maintaining a control environment that sets a positive attitude toward internal control and conscientious management, including an organizational structure with clearly defined areas of authority and responsibility. See GAO, Standards for Internal Control in the Federal Government, GAO/AIMD-00-21.3.1 (Washington, D.C.: November 1999), and Internal Control Management and Evaluation Tool, GAO-01-1008G (Washington, D.C.: August 2001).

[10] The other reserve categories are the Individual Ready Reserve, Standby Reserve, and Retired Reserve.

[11] According to officials, this number is not the official strength of the Selected Reserve.

[12] See Pub. L. No. 108-375, § 701, 118 Stat. 1811, 1980-82 (2004).

[13] See Pub. L. No. 109-163, §§ 701-702, 119 Stat. 3136, 3339-42 (2006); Pub. L. No. 109-364, § 706, 120 Stat. 2083, 2282 (2006).

[14] For example, the NDAA for Fiscal Year 2009 specified that the appropriate actuarial basis for calculating TRS premiums should utilize the actual cost of providing benefits to TRS members and their dependents in preceding calendar years beginning with calendar year 2010.

[15] A contingency operation is a military operation that is designated by the Secretary of Defense as an operation in which members of the Armed Forces are or may become involved in military actions, operations, or hostilities against an enemy of the United States or against an opposing force or a military operation that results in the call-up to (or retention on) active duty of members of the uniformed Services under certain statutes during war or a national emergency declared by the President or Congress.

[16] For tier one, a reservist must have had qualifying active duty service in support of a contingency operation on or after September 11, 2001, for at least 90 days and must have agreed to serve in the Selected Reserve for the entire period of TRS coverage. The reservist must have executed this service agreement within 90 days after release from active duty. The reservist was responsible for paying 28 percent of the premium. For tier two a reservist who did not qualify for tier one must not have been eligible for employer-sponsored health insurance, or must have been eligible for unemployment compensation, or must have been self-employed, and must have executed a service agreement to serve in the Selected Reserve for the entire period of TRS coverage. The reservist must have qualified during open season or submitted documentation establishing a qualifying life event. The reservist was responsible for paying 50 percent of the premium. For tier three, a reservist who did not qualify for tier one or two may have been eligible for employer-sponsored insurance, but must have executed a service agreement to serve in the Selected Reserve for the entire period of TRS coverage. The reservist must have qualified during open season or submitted documentation establishing a qualifying life event. The reservist was responsible for paying 85 percent of the premium.

[17] The NDAA for Fiscal Year 2008, provided that certain members of the Selected Reserve, who were eligible for the FEHB Program, could continue to receive benefits under their previous tier 1 TRS agreement despite FEHB eligibility.

[18] Retirees and certain dependents and survivors who are entitled to Medicare Part A and enrolled in Part B, and who are generally age 65 and older, are eligible to obtain care under a separate program called TRICARE for Life. TRICARE for Life is a program that supplements Medicare coverage for Medicare-eligible beneficiaries enrolled in Medicare Part B. TRICARE beneficiaries under 65 years of age who are eligible for Medicare Part A

on the basis of disability or end-stage renal disease are eligible for TRICARE for Life if they enroll in Medicare Part B.

[19] For members activated not in support of a contingency operation, TRICARE coverage becomes effective when active duty starts.

[20] Members activated not in support of a contingency operation are not eligible for the Transitional Assistance Management Program and return to inactive status immediately after returning from active duty.

[21] The current managed care support contracts are the second generation of TRICARE contracts and the implementation period for these contracts was set to end on March 31, 2010, with the third generation of contracts to begin on April 1, 2010. However, this timeline was delayed because of to bid protests on two of the three contracts.

[22] Prime Service Areas are determined by the Assistant Secretary of Defense for Health Affairs and are defined by a set of five-digit zip codes, usually within an approximate 40- mile radius of a military inpatient treatment facility. However, the contractors were allowed to offer expanded or additional Prime Service Areas beyond the 40-mile radius.

[23] A unit commander exercises authority over subordinates within a unit by virtue of rank or assignment. A commander has the authority and responsibility for effectively using available resources and for planning the employment of, organizing, directing, coordinating, and controlling military forces for the accomplishment of assigned missions. Within the reserve components, the unit under the control of the commander can consist of any number of servicemembers organized hierarchically into groups of various sizes for functional, tactical, and administrative purposes.

[24] Officials from a second reserve component stated that they have a staff member who maintains information on a Web site about TRICARE; however, this person does not serve as a central point of contact for TRS education.

[25] This survey was based on the Health Care Survey of Department of Defense Beneficiaries, which was designed to provide a comprehensive look at beneficiary opinions about their DOD health care benefits. Members of the Selected Reserve are included in this survey. Officials told us that over time they have analyzed responses from members of the Selected Reserve and these responses were the impetus behind conducting this focused survey in 2008. TMA officials are currently repeating the Focused Survey of TRICARE Reserve Select and Selected Reserve Military Health System Access and Satisfaction.

[26] Department of Defense, TRICARE Management Activity, Evaluation of the TRICARE Program: Fiscal Year 2009 Report to Congress (Washington D.C., 2009).

[27] Access to more affordable civilian options and opportunities to obtain civilian health insurance also affected the decision not to enroll.

[28] GAO, Human Capital: Quality of DOD Status of Forces Surveys Could Be Improved by Performing Nonresponse Analysis of the Results, GAO-10-751R (Washington, D.C.: July 12, 2010).

[29] GAO, Defense Health Care: Access to Civilian Providers under TRICARE Standard and Extra, GAO-11-500 (Washington, D.C.: June 2, 2011).

[30] For additional information on how TMA generally addressed the methodological requirements, see GAO, Defense Health Care: 2008 Access to Care Surveys Indicate Some Problems, but Beneficiary Satisfaction Is Similar to Other Health Plans, GAO-10-402 (Washington, D.C.: Mar. 31, 2010).

[31] For the purpose of this analysis, claims consist of all services provided by a professional, including a doctor or nurse, and do not include services submitted by an institution. In addition, these claims do not include inpatient care, medical supplies, or pharmacy claims.

[32] Allergic rhinitis is a collection of symptoms, mostly in the nose and eyes, which occur when a person breathes in something the person is allergic to, such as dust, dander, or pollen.

[33] These percentages include members of the Selected Reserve and their dependents. Selected Reserve members living overseas, in unknown locations, and in Puerto Rico and Guam were not included in this analysis.

End Note for Appendix I

[1] Claims filed for fiscal year 2010 may not be complete because individuals have up to 1 year to file a claim.

In: Military Health Care
Editor: Brian M. Gagliardi

ISBN: 978-1-62417-339-4
© 2013 Nova Science Publishers, Inc.

Chapter 4

DEFENSE HEALTH CARE: ACCESS TO CIVILIAN PROVIDERS UNDER TRICARE STANDARD AND EXTRA[*]

United States Government Accountability Office

ABBREVIATIONS

BRAC	Base Realignment and Closure
CPT	current procedural terminology
DOD	Department of Defense
NDAA	National Defense Authorization Act
PPACA	Patient Protection and Affordable Care Act
TMA	TRICARE Management Activity

WHY GAO DID THIS STUDY

The Department of Defense (DOD) provides health care through its TRICARE program, which is managed by the TRICARE Management Activity (TMA). TRICARE offers three basic options. Beneficiaries who

---

[*] This is an edited, reformatted and augmented version of The United States Government Accountability Office publication, Report to Congressional Committees GAO-11-500, dated June 2011.

choose TRICARE Prime, an option that uses civilian provider networks, must enroll. TRICARE beneficiaries who do not enroll in this option may obtain care from nonnetwork providers under TRICARE Standard or from network providers under TRICARE Extra.

The National Defense Authorization Act for Fiscal Year 2008 directed GAO to evaluate various aspects of beneficiaries' access to care under the TRICARE Standard and Extra options. This report examines (1) impediments to TRICARE Standard and Extra beneficiaries' access to civilian health care and mental health care providers and TMA's actions to address the impediments; (2) TMA's efforts to monitor access to civilian providers for TRICARE Standard and Extra beneficiaries; (3) how TMA informs network and nonnetwork civilian providers about TRICARE Standard and Extra; and (4) how TMA informs TRICARE Standard and Extra beneficiaries about their options. To address these objectives, GAO reviewed and analyzed TMA and TRICARE contractor data and documents. GAO also interviewed TMA officials, including those in its regional offices, as well as its contractors.

WHAT GAO FOUND

Reimbursement rates and provider shortages have been cited as the main impediments that hinder TRICARE Standard and Extra beneficiaries' access to civilian health care and mental health care providers. Providers' concern about TRICARE's reimbursement rates—which are generally set at Medicare rates—has been a long-standing issue and has more recently been cited as the primary reason civilian providers will not accept TRICARE Standard and Extra beneficiaries as patients, according to TMA's surveys of civilian providers. TMA can increase reimbursement rates in certain instances, such as when it determines that access to care is being affected by the level of reimbursement. Shortages of certain provider specialties, such as mental health care providers, at the national and local levels may also impede access, but these shortages are not specific to the TRICARE program and also affect the general population. As a result, there are limitations as to what TMA can do to address them.

TMA has primarily used feedback mechanisms, including surveys of beneficiaries and civilian providers, to gauge TRICARE Standard and Extra beneficiaries' access to civilian providers. More recently, in February 2010, in recognition that TRICARE has had no established measures for monitoring the availability of civilian network and nonnetwork providers for these beneficiaries, TMA directed the TRICARE Regional Offices to develop a model to help identify geographic areas where they may experience access problems. GAO's review of the initial models found their methodology to be reasonable. However, because the regional models were recently developed, it is too early to determine their effectiveness.

TMA's contractors educate civilian providers about TRICARE program requirements, policies, and procedures. Contractors also conduct outreach to increase providers' awareness of the program, and while TMA's provider survey results indicate that civilian providers are generally aware of the program, this does not necessarily signify that providers have an accurate understanding of the TRICARE program and its options.

Similarly, TMA's contractors educate beneficiaries on all of the TRICARE options and maintain directories of network providers to facilitate beneficiaries' access to care. When the new TRICARE contracts are implemented, TMA will also require its contractors to include information on nonnetwork providers in their provider directories.

In commenting on a draft of this report, DOD concurred with GAO's overall findings.

June 2, 2011

The Honorable Carl Levin
Chairman

The Honorable John McCain
Ranking Member
Committee on Armed Services
United States Senate

The Honorable Howard P. "Buck" McKeon
Chairman

The Honorable Adam Smith
Ranking Member
Committee on Armed Services
House of Representatives

In fiscal year 2010, the Department of Defense (DOD) offered health care to almost 9.7 million eligible beneficiaries through its TRICARE program.[1] Under TRICARE, beneficiaries may choose among three basic options— TRICARE Prime (a managed care option), TRICARE Extra (a preferred provider organization option), and TRICARE Standard (a fee-for-service option).[2] TRICARE is different from other health care plans because not all of the options require eligible beneficiaries to enroll to use their benefits. Beneficiaries who choose TRICARE Prime are required to enroll in this option. Beneficiaries who decide not to use TRICARE Prime may still obtain health care through the TRICARE program by using either the TRICARE Standard or Extra options, or they may choose not to use their TRICARE benefits at all.[3] Consequently, DOD does not have complete information on which beneficiaries intend to use their benefits, and it cannot accurately predict the health care demands of beneficiaries who have not enrolled, including how to ensure adequate access to care.

Under TRICARE, beneficiaries can obtain care either from providers at military hospitals and clinics, referred to as military treatment facilities, or from civilian providers. DOD's TRICARE Management Activity (TMA), which oversees the program, contracts with managed care support contractors (contractors) to develop networks of civilian providers and to perform other customer service functions, such as processing claims and assisting beneficiaries with finding providers. Contractors are required to establish adequate networks of civilian providers to serve all TRICARE beneficiaries regardless of enrollment status in geographic areas called Prime Service Areas.[4] Contractors use estimates of the number of TRICARE users, among other factors, to develop provider networks and ensure adequate access to care for beneficiaries. Although some network providers may be located outside of Prime Service Areas, contractors are not required to develop networks in these areas (which we refer to as non-Prime Service Areas).

All beneficiaries may obtain care at military treatment facilities, although priority is given to active duty personnel and then to beneficiaries enrolled in TRICARE Prime. Beneficiaries who enroll in TRICARE Prime can also obtain care from the civilian providers who have joined the provider network established by the TRICARE contractors—referred to as network providers.[5] Beneficiaries who do not enroll in TRICARE Prime may receive care either from network providers, in which case they are considered to be using TRICARE Extra, or from nonnetwork providers (those outside the network), in which case they are considered to be using TRICARE Standard. The choices that beneficiaries have in selecting TRICARE options and providers vary depending on their location. Beneficiaries living in Prime Service Areas can choose between TRICARE Prime, TRICARE Standard, and TRICARE Extra. Beneficiaries living in non-PrimeService Areas can choose between TRICARE Standard and TRICARE Extra. According to a TMA official, about 19 percent of beneficiaries eligible for TRICARE Standard and Extra resided in non-Prime Service Areas in fiscal year 2010.

Since TRICARE's inception in 1995, beneficiaries using the TRICARE Standard and Extra options have reported difficulties finding civilian providers who will accept them as patients. In response to these concerns, the National Defense Authorization Act (NDAA) for Fiscal Year 2004 directed DOD to monitor access to care for TRICARE beneficiaries who were not enrolled in TRICARE Prime through a multiyear survey of civilian providers.[6] According to TMA, which administered the survey, results indicated that nationally, about 81 percent of physicians who were accepting new patients would accept TRICARE beneficiaries as patients, although the results varied by state and by provider specialty. The act also directed us to review the processes, procedures, and analysis used by DOD to determine the adequacy of the number of network and nonnetwork civilian providers and the actions DOD has taken to ensure access to care for beneficiaries who were not enrolled in TRICARE Prime. In December 2006, we reported that TMA and its contractors used various methods to monitor access to care, and these methods indicated that access was generally sufficient for users of TRICARE Standard and Extra.[7]

Nonetheless, beneficiaries using the TRICARE Standard and Extra options have continued to express concerns about access to civilian providers. To better understand the adequacy of access to care for this population, the NDAA for Fiscal Year 2008 directed DOD to conduct two surveys[8]— another multiyear survey of civilian providers as well as a multiyear survey of beneficiaries, which includes nonenrolled beneficiaries who were eligible to use the TRICARE Standard and TRICARE Extra options as well as TRICARE Reserve Select—an option similar to TRICARE Standard and Extra that is available to certain members of the Reserves and National Guard. The NDAA for Fiscal Year 2008 directed us to review these surveys, and in March 2010, we reported that the methodology for DOD's surveys of civilian providers and nonenrolled beneficiaries was sound, and we provided an analysis of the first year's results for each of the surveys.[9]

Furthermore, access to mental health care providers is of particular concern for all TRICARE beneficiaries, including those who use TRICARE Standard and Extra, because the exposure to combat and the stress of deployment and redeployment have increased beneficiaries' demand for mental health services. From fiscal year 2006 through 2010, TRICARE Standard and Extra beneficiaries' visits to civilian mental health care providers increased over 27 percent. A June 2007 report by DOD's Task Force on Mental Health stated that TRICARE's provider networks have been tasked with providing an increasing volume and proportion of mental health services for families and retirees.[10] In assessing the oversight of the mental health network at one location, the task force discovered that out of 100 network mental health providers contacted from a list on the contractor's Web site, only 3 would accept new TRICARE patients.

The NDAA for Fiscal Year 2008 directed us to evaluate issues related to TRICARE Standard and Extra beneficiaries' access to health care and mental health care, including the identification of access impediments and education and outreach efforts directed at civilian providers and these beneficiaries. This report identifies and examines: (1) the impediments to TRICARE Standard and Extra beneficiaries' access to civilian health care and mental health care providers and TMA's actions to address the impediments; (2) TMA's efforts to monitor access to civilian providers for TRICARE Standard and Extra beneficiaries; (3) how TMA informs network and nonnetwork civilian providers about TRICARE Standard and Extra; and (4) how TMA informs TRICARE Standard and Extra beneficiaries about their options and facilitates their access to network and nonnetwork civilian providers.

To address these objectives, we met with officials in each of the three TRICARE Regional Offices (North, South, and West) and with officials for each of the three contractors to discuss access impediments in their respective regions, how access to network and nonnetwork providers is monitored, and their efforts to educate civilian providers and TRICARE Standard and Extra beneficiaries. We also interviewed TMA officials responsible for program operations, medical benefits and reimbursement, contract performance evaluation, contract management, data quality, communication and customer service, and program analysis and evaluation. We also obtained documentation on the contractors' performance in meeting network adequacy and education related requirements. Lastly, we met with representatives of military beneficiary organizations as well as two national provider organizations to obtain their perspectives about access to civilian providers for TRICARE Standard and Extra beneficiaries.

To identify and examine impediments to TRICARE Standard and Extra beneficiaries' access to civilian health care and mental health care providers and TMA's actions to address them, we obtained and reviewed relevant reports and studies. Specifically, we reviewed TMA's reported results from its multiyear survey of civilian providers, conducted from 2005 through 2007, as well as the first 2 years of its subsequent surveys of these providers during fiscal years 2008 and 2009. We assessed the reliability of these data by speaking with knowledgeable officials and reviewing related documentation, and we determined that the survey results were sufficiently reliable for the purposes of this report. We also reviewed a 2008 report prepared by CNA[11] on the current participation of civilian providers in the TRICARE program. To examine how TMA addresses access impediments, we reviewed TMA's reimbursement policies, studies that assessed TRICARE's reimbursement rates, TMA's procedures for increasing reimbursement rates, and TMA's procedures for offering bonus payments to physicians in areas identified as having physician shortages. We obtained TMA's reported data on adjustments to reimbursement rates that it issued between January 2002 and January 2011. However, we did not assess the appropriateness of TMA's decision to make these adjustments or the extent to which these adjustments improved civilian providers' acceptance of TRICARE beneficiaries as patients. Additionally, we reviewed DOD's 2009 Report to Congress: Access to Mental Health Services, and spoke with TMA and contractor officials about access to mental health care and actions to improve access.

To identify and examine the mechanisms that TMA uses to monitor TRICARE Standard and Extra beneficiaries' access to civilian providers, we reviewed various efforts, including feedback mechanisms, that TMA and its contractors use to solicit and gauge beneficiaries' concerns, including difficulties with access to civilian providers. These feedback mechanisms included TMA's surveys of civilian providers and nonenrolled beneficiaries (TRICARE Standard, TRICARE Extra, and TRICARE Reserve Select), as well as data collected on beneficiaries' inquiries and complaints by TMA and its contractors during either fiscal or calendar years 2008 through 2010. We spoke with TMA officials and obtained information from its contractors about the reliability of their data on beneficiaries' inquiries and determined them to be sufficiently reliable for the purpose of our report, but we did not independently verify these data. We also reviewed TMA's 2010 memorandum that directed the TRICARE Regional Offices to implement a new approach for monitoring access to civilian providers under the TRICARE Standard and Extra options, and we obtained and reviewed information about each regional office's monitoring methodology.

To identify and examine how TMA informs network and nonnetwork civilian providers and beneficiaries about TRICARE Standard and Extra and how it facilitates access to civilian providers, we reviewed TMA's requirements of its contractors as related to educating providers and beneficiaries in each TRICARE region under the second generation of TRICARE managed care support contracts (contracts).[12] We also reviewed each contractor's marketing and education plans to identify their specific education efforts. Additionally, we obtained and reviewed TRICARE provider and beneficiary educational materials to gain an understanding of the information that TMA and the contractors use to educate providers and beneficiaries. However, we did not assess the quality and effectiveness of TMA's or the contractors' education efforts and materials. Finally, we reviewed TMA's 2010 memorandum and related documentation regarding TMA's effort to facilitate access to care through provider directories for TRICARE Standard and Extra beneficiaries.

We conducted this performance audit from July 2010 through June 2011 in accordance with generally accepted government auditing standards. Those standards require that we plan and perform the audit to obtain sufficient, appropriate evidence to provide a reasonable basis for our findings based on our audit objectives. We believe that the evidence obtained provides a reasonable basis for our findings and conclusions based on our audit objectives.

BACKGROUND

In fiscal year 2010, DOD offered health care to almost 9.7 million eligible beneficiaries through its TRICARE program. TRICARE is organized into three regions, and within these regions, beneficiaries may obtain health care from either providers at military treatment facilities or civilian providers.

TRICARE's Benefit Options

TRICARE provides three basic options for its non-Medicare-eligible beneficiary population. These options vary according to TRICARE beneficiary enrollment requirements, the choices TRICARE beneficiaries have in selecting civilian and military treatment facility providers and the amount TRICARE beneficiaries must contribute towards the cost of their care. (See table 1.)

Table 1. Summary of TRICARE's Basic Options

TRICARE option	Description
TRICARE Prime	Beneficiaries who choose to use this managed care option must enroll. All active duty servicemembers are required to use TRICARE Prime, but other TRICARE eligible (i.e., non-active duty) beneficiaries may choose to use this option and must enroll to do so. TRICARE Prime enrollees may pay an annual enrollment fee[a] and receive most of their care from providers at military treatment facilities, augmented by network providers who have agreed to meet specific standards for appointment wait times among other requirements. TRICARE Prime offers lower out-of-pocket costs than the other TRICARE options.
TRICARE Standard	TRICARE beneficiaries who choose not to enroll in TRICARE Prime may obtain health care from nonnetwork providers. Under this option, beneficiaries must pay an annual deductible and cost-shares, which vary among active duty dependents and retirees and their dependents. There is no annual enrollment fee.
TRICARE Extra	Similar to TRICARE Standard, beneficiaries do not have to enroll or pay an annual enrollment fee for TRICARE Extra. Under this option, beneficiaries may obtain care from a TRICARE network civilian provider for lower cost-shares (about 5 percentage points less) than they would have if they saw nonnetwork providers under the TRICARE Standard option.

Source: GAO summary of the Department of Defense's TRICARE documentation.
Note: All beneficiaries may obtain care at military treatment facilities although priority
   is given to any active-duty personnel and then to TRICARE Prime enrollees.
[a]There is no annual enrollment fee for active duty servicemembers and their
   dependents. However, retirees and their dependents under 65 years must pay an
   annual enrollment fee.

TRICARE also offers other options, including TRICARE Reserve Select, a premium-based health plan that certain Reserve and National Guard servicemembers may purchase. Under TRICARE Reserve Select, beneficiaries may obtain health care from either nonnetwork or network providers, similar to beneficiaries using TRICARE Standard or Extra, respectively, and pay lower cost-shares for using network providers.

TRICARE Regional Structure and Contracts

TRICARE is a regionally structured program that is organized into three main regions—North, South, and West. (See fig. 1 for the location of the three regions.) TMA manages civilian health care in each of these regions through contractors. As of March 2011, the second generation of TRICARE contracts were in operation, and TMA was in the process of awarding the third generation of contracts.

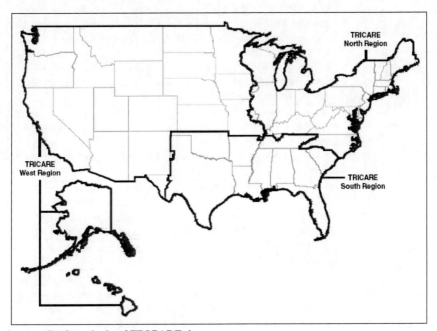

Source: GAO analysis of TRICARE data.

Figure 1. Location of TRICARE Regions.

The contractors are required to establish and maintain adequate networks of civilian providers within designated locations referred to as Prime Service Areas. In these areas, civilian provider networks are required to be large enough to provide access for all TRICARE beneficiaries, regardless of enrollment status or Medicare eligibility. These civilian provider networks are also required to meet specific access standards for TRICARE Prime beneficiaries—such as for travel times or wait times.[13] However the access standards do not apply to beneficiaries using options other than TRICARE Prime, such as TRICARE Standard or Extra. The contractors are also responsible for helping TRICARE beneficiaries locate providers and for informing and educating TRICARE beneficiaries and providers on all aspects of the TRICARE program. In addition, they provide customer service to any

TRICARE beneficiary who requests assistance, regardless of their enrollment status.

TMA has a TRICARE Regional Office in each region that helps to manage health care delivery. These offices are responsible for overseeing the contractors, including monitoring network quality and adequacy and customer-satisfaction outcomes. Similar to the contractors' efforts, these offices provide customer service to all TRICARE beneficiaries who request assistance, regardless of their enrollment status.

TRICARE Network and Nonnetwork Civilian Providers

Civilian providers must be TRICARE-authorized to be reimbursed for care under the program.[14] Such authorization requires a provider to be licensed by their state, accredited by a national organization, if one exists, and meet other standards of the medical community. There are two types of authorized civilian providers—network and nonnetwork providers, and both types of providers may accept TRICARE beneficiaries as patients on a case-by-case basis, regardless of enrollment status.

- *Network providers* are TRICARE-authorized providers who enter into a contract with the regional contractor to provide care to TRICARE beneficiaries and agree to accept TRICARE reimbursement rates as payment in full.[15] By law, TRICARE reimbursement rates for civilian providers are generally limited to Medicare rates, but network providers may agree to accept lower reimbursements as a condition of network membership.[16] Network providers are not obligated to accept all TRICARE beneficiaries seeking care. For example, network providers may decline to accept TRICARE beneficiaries as patients because their practices do not have sufficient capacity or for other reasons.[17]
- *Nonnetwork providers* are TRICARE-authorized providers who have not entered into a contractual agreement with a contractor to provide care to TRICARE beneficiaries. Nonnetwork providers may accept the TRICARE reimbursement rate as payment in full or they may charge up to 15 percent above the reimbursement amount. The beneficiary is responsible for paying the extra amount billed in addition to the required cost-shares.

Beneficiaries' Use of TRICARE

Claims data from fiscal years 2006 through 2010 show that overall TRICARE claims paid to civilian providers have increased by more than 50 percent, even though the eligible population increased by less than 6 percent.[18] (See table 2.)

Table 2. TRICARE-eligible Beneficiaries and Claims Paid to Civilian Providers for Fiscal Years 2006 through 2010

Fiscal year	TRICARE-eligible beneficiaries (million)[a]	TRICARE claims paid to civilian providers (million)
2006	9.19	19.29
2007	9.22	21.31
2008	9.39	24.02
2009	9.58	26.97
2010	9.69	29.60[b]
Total percentage change from fiscal year 2006 to 2010	5.4 percent	53.4 percent

Source: GAO analysis of TRICARE Management Activity (TMA) data.

Note: Claims were for services provided in an office or other setting outside of an institution. Claims for services rendered at hospitals, military treatment facilities, and other institutions were excluded.

TRICARE for Life claims were excluded as well as claims for medical supplies and from chiropractors and pharmacies.

[a] Eligible beneficiaries include active duty personnel and their dependents, medically eligible Reserve and National Guard personnel and their dependents, and retirees and their dependents and survivors.

[b] Fiscal year 2010 data are incomplete as TMA allows claims to be submitted up to 1 year after care was provided.

Between fiscal years 2006 through 2010, TRICARE Standard and Extra beneficiaries' use of network providers—as measured by the number of claims paid to network providers—has increased significantly, while their use of nonnetwork providers—as measured by the number of claims paid to nonnetwork providers—has slightly decreased. (See fig. 2.) Specifically, their use of network providers has increased more than 66 percent between fiscal years 2006 and 2010, compared to about a 10 percent decrease in the use of nonnetwork providers over the same time period.

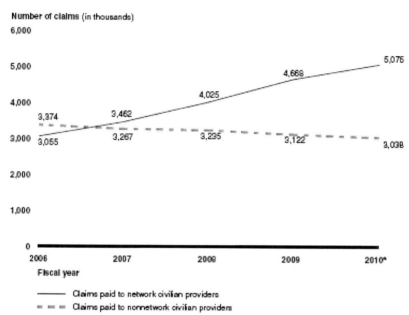

Number of claims (in thousands)

Source: GAO analysis of TRICARE Management Activity (TMA) data.

Note: Claims analyzed were for services provided in an office or other setting outside of an institution. Claims for services rendered at hospitals, military treatment facilities, and other institutions were excluded. TRICARE for Life claims were excluded as well as claims for medical supplies and from chiropractors and pharmacies.

[a] Fiscal year 2010 data are incomplete as TMA allows claims to be submitted up to 1 year after care was provided.

Figure 2. TRICARE Standard and Extra Beneficiaries' Claims Paid to Network and Nonnetwork Civilian Providers for Fiscal Years 2006 Through 2010.

REIMBURSEMENT RATES AND PROVIDER SHORTAGES HINDER ACCESS TO CIVILIAN PROVIDERS; TMA CAN INCREASE REIMBURSEMENT RATES WHEN NEEDED, BUT HAS ONLY LIMITED MEANS TO ADDRESS SHORTAGES

Reimbursement rates have been cited as the primary impediment that hinders beneficiaries' access to civilian health care and mental health care providers under TRICARE Standard and Extra. TMA can increase reimbursement rates in certain circumstances when a need has been demonstrated. Although national and local shortages of certain types of providers have also been cited as an impediment to TRICARE Standard and Extra beneficiaries' access to civilian providers, TMA is limited in its ability to address this impediment as it affects the general population and not just TRICARE beneficiaries. Additionally, beneficiaries' access to mental health care is affected by provider shortages and other issues and is of particular concern because the stress of deployment and redeployment has increased the demand for these services.

Reimbursement Rates Have Been Cited as the Primary Impediment to Beneficiaries' Access to Civilian Providers under TRICARE Standard and Extra, and TMA Can Adjust Them When a Need is Demonstrated

Since TRICARE was implemented in 1995, some civilian providers—both network and nonnetwork—have expressed concerns about TRICARE's reimbursement rates. For example, in 2006, we reported that both network and nonnetwork civilian providers said that TRICARE's reimbursement rates tended to be lower than those of other health plans, and as a result, some of these providers had been unwilling to accept TRICARE Standard and Extra beneficiaries as patients.[19] More recent studies by TMA and others have cited TRICARE's reimbursement rates as the primary reason civilian providers may be unwilling to accept these beneficiaries as patients, for example:

- TMA's first multiyear survey of civilian providers (2005 through 2007) showed that TRICARE's reimbursement rates were the primary reason cited by providers for not accepting TRICARE Standard and Extra beneficiaries as new patients.[20]
- Similarly, results from the first 2 years (2008 and 2009) of TMA's second multiyear provider survey showed that the responding providers cited TRICARE's reimbursement rates as one of the primary reasons that they would not accept new TRICARE patients even though they would accept new Medicare patients.[21]
- In a 2008 study on civilian providers' acceptance of TRICARE Standard and Extra beneficiaries, CNA reported that the medical society officials and physicians they interviewed cited low reimbursement as the primary reason for limiting their acceptance of TRICARE beneficiaries as patients.[22] The providers who were

interviewed as part of this study noted that while they could accept more TRICARE beneficiaries as patients, there are services for which the reimbursement was so low that accepting more TRICARE beneficiaries as patients hurt rather than helped them.

In addition to these studies, officials from each of the TRICARE Regional Offices and two of the contractors, as well as a national provider organization, told us that reimbursement rates were civilian providers' primary concern about TRICARE.

Concerns about TRICARE's reimbursement rates—which generally mirror the Medicare program's physician fee schedule23—have increased by the uncertainty surrounding the annual update to these Medicare fees.24 All of the contractors expressed concerns about the proposed decreases to Medicare rates and how that would affect providers' acceptance of TRICARE patients. One contractor told us that providers already were expressing concerns about the Medicare rate decreases and that some providers said they would no longer accept TRICARE beneficiaries as patients if the rates were reduced. Furthermore, as of September 2010, this contractor noted that one provider had stopped accepting TRICARE beneficiaries as patients because of concerns about potential Medicare reimbursement reductions.

TMA has the authority to adjust TRICARE reimbursement rates under certain conditions to increase beneficiaries' access to civilian providers, and has done so in some instances. In response to various concerns about providers' willingness to accept TRICARE patients, TMA contracted with a consulting firm to conduct a number of studies about TRICARE reimbursement rates, and some of these studies have resulted in increases to reimbursement amounts for certain procedures. (See app. II for a summary of the studies.) For example, in response to civilian obstetric providers' concerns about TRICARE reimbursement rates, TMA conducted an analysis of historical TRICARE claims data and made nationwide changes to its physician payment rates for obstetric care in 2006.25 These changes included an additional payment for ultrasounds for uncomplicated pregnancies that is likely to result in overall higher payments for civilian physicians who perform one or more ultrasounds during the course of pregnancy.

TMA also has the authority to adjust reimbursement rates through the use of waivers in areas where it determines that the rates have had a negative impact on TRICARE beneficiaries' access to civilian providers. TMA can issue three types of reimbursement waivers, depending on the type of adjustment that is needed:

- Locality waivers may be used to increase rates for specific medical services in specific areas where access to civilian providers has been severely impaired and are applicable to both network and nonnetwork providers.[26]
- Network waivers may be used to increase reimbursement rates for network providers up to 15 percent above the TRICARE reimbursement rate in an effort to ensure an adequate number and mix of primary and specialty care network civilian providers in a specific location.[27]
- TMA can restore TRICARE reimbursement rates in specific localities to the levels that existed before a reduction was made to align TRICARE reimbursement rates with Medicare rates for both network and nonnetwork providers.[28]

Waivers can be requested by providers, beneficiaries, contractors, military treatment facilities, or TRICARE Regional Office directors, although all requests must be submitted through the TRICARE Regional Office directors. Individuals may apply for waivers by submitting written requests to the TRICARE Regional Offices.

These requests must contain specific justifications to support the claim that access problems are related to low reimbursement rates and must include information such as the number of providers and TRICARE-eligible beneficiaries in a location, the availability of military treatment facility providers, geographic characteristics, and the cost-effectiveness of granting the waiver.

Ultimately, the TRICARE Regional Office director reviews and analyzes the requests.

If the TRICARE Regional Office director agrees with the request, they make a recommendation to the Director of TMA that the waiver request be approved. Each analysis is tailored to the specific concerns outlined in the waiver requests.

Once implemented, waivers remain in effect indefinitely or until TMA officials determine they are no longer needed.

As shown in table 3, the total number of waivers has increased from 15 to 24 since we last reported on TMA's use of waivers in 2006. (See app. III for more details about the waivers.)

Additionally, 13 of the 24 waivers are for locations in Alaska. (See app. IV for more information about access-tocare issues in Alaska.)

**Table 3. TRICARE Reimbursement Waivers in August 2006
and January 2011**

Type of waiver	Number of waivers in place as of August 2006	Number of waivers in place as of January 2011
Locality waiver	7	16
Network waiver	6	8
Waiving reimbursement rate reductionsa	2	0
Total	15	24

Source: GAO analysis of TRICARE Management Activity (TMA) data.

aTMA has authority to restore TRICARE reimbursement rates in specific localities to the levels that existed before a reduction was made to align TRICARE reimbursement rates with Medicare rates. The two waivers that were in place in 2006 were for Alaska and were discontinued when a demonstration project, implemented in 2007, increased TRICARE's reimbursement rates so that on average, they matched those of the Department of Veterans Affairs.

Other than assessing the effectiveness of a specific rate adjustment in Alaska, TMA has not conducted analyses to determine if its rate adjustments or the use of waivers have increased beneficiaries' access to civilian providers. Nonetheless, officials told us that using the waivers has proved to be successful by maintaining the stability of the provider networks and by increasing the size of the networks in some areas.

National and Local Shortages of Certain Provider Specialties Impede Beneficiaries' Access to Civilian Providers, and TMA Is Limited in Its Ability to Address Them

Another main impediment to TRICARE beneficiaries' access to civilian providers is a shortage of certain provider specialties, both at the national and local levels. However, TMA is limited in its ability to address provider shortages because this impediment affects the entire health care delivery system and is not specific to the TRICARE program.

National and Local Shortages of Certain Provider Specialties
Impede Access

Although the number of civilian providers accepting TRICARE has increased over the years,[29] access to civilian providers remains a concern due to national and local shortages of certain provider specialties. These shortages limit access for the general population, including all TRICARE beneficiaries regardless of enrollment status. Several organizations have reported on national provider work-force shortages in primary care as well as in a number of specialties.[30] For example, the Association of American Medical Colleges reported national shortages in provider specialties such as anesthesiology, dermatology, and psychiatry. Additionally, the contractors and regional office officials we met with told us that they were particularly concerned about the national shortage of child psychiatrists.

In addition to national shortages, TRICARE beneficiaries' access to civilian providers also may be impeded in certain locations where there are insufficient numbers and types of civilian providers to cover the local demand for health care. According to the contractors, each TRICARE region had areas with civilian provider shortages, for example:

- In TRICARE's West region, a Prime Service Area in northern California had provider shortages in 21 different provider specialties, including allergists and obstetricians as well as psychologists and psychiatrists. According to this region's contractor, either there were no providers located in the area or the providers located in the area were already contracted as TRICARE network providers.
- In TRICARE's South region, the contractor identified locations in Texas, Louisiana, and Florida in which there were limited numbers of specialists and mental health providers. For example, according to this contractor, Del Rio, Texas has no providers in several specialties including dermatology, allergy, and psychiatry.
- Likewise, in TRICARE's North region, the contractor stated that there are mountainous areas, such as parts of West Virginia, and remote areas, such as western North Carolina, in which there are provider shortages. Consequently, the general population, including TRICARE beneficiaries, has to drive longer distances to obtain certain types of specialty care.

TMA is Limited in How it Can Address Provider Shortages

TMA has attempted to address civilian provider shortages, but because these shortages are not specific to the TRICARE program, there are limitations in what TMA can do. One step TMA has taken is the adoption of a bonus payment system that mirrors the one used by Medicare for certain provider shortage areas.[31] Under Medicare, providers who provide services to beneficiaries located in Health Professional Shortage Areas— geographic areas that the Department of Health and Human Services has identified as having shortages of primary health, dental, or mental health care providers— receive 10 percent bonus payments.[32] Beginning in June 2003, TMA began offering providers a 10 percent bonus payment for services rendered in these same locations. TMA estimated that from fiscal year 2007 through the third quarter of fiscal year 2010, more than 20,000 individual providers received these payments.

Currently, civilian providers must include a specific code on every TRICARE claim they submit to obtain the additional payment. However, TMA officials noted that some providers may not be receiving this bonus because they do not include the specific code on their claims. TMA officials noted the process will become easier once the third generation of managed care support contracts is implemented. Once this occurs, the contractors will rely on the Centers for Medicare & Medicaid Services' public database of zip codes to determine a provider's eligibility for these bonus payments instead of requiring the provider to include a code on each claim. TMA officials estimated that this change will result in an additional $150,000 in bonus payments each year for TRICARE claims.

TRICARE Beneficiaries' Access to Mental Health Care Is Affected by Provider Shortages and Other Issues

Access to mental health care is a concern for all TRICARE beneficiaries, and it has been affected by provider shortages and other issues, including providers' lack of knowledge about combat related issues, providers' concerns about reimbursement rates, and providers' lack of awareness about TRICARE. A 2007 report by the American Psychological Association noted that shortages of mental health providers specifically trained in military issues and the challenge associated with modifying the military culture so that mental health services are less stigmatized are impediments to TRICARE beneficiaries' access to mental health care.[33] Furthermore, the report discusses that even where mental health providers are available, it can be difficult to find psychiatrists and other mental health providers with specific familiarity of TRICARE beneficiaries' mental health conditions such as post-traumatic stress disorder and deployment issues. This can be frustrating for TRICARE beneficiaries who seek mental health care only to discover that providers cannot relate to their specific concerns.

Over the years, Congress has required DOD to report on TRICARE beneficiaries' access to mental health care providers. Specifically, the NDAA for Fiscal Year 2008 required DOD to report on the adequacy of access to mental health services under the TRICARE program. In 2009, DOD reported that it believed access to mental health care providers for TRICARE beneficiaries was adequate due to a dramatic increase in both inpatient and outpatient mental health care provided in 2008.[34] DOD also cited increases in the numbers of mental health providers from May 2007 to May 2009 in both the direct care system of military treatment facilities (1,952) and in the civilian provider network (10,220), while acknowledging that there may still be some areas where access to mental health care providers is inadequate. However, in the same report, DOD noted that TRICARE Standard and Extra beneficiaries reported more problems finding civilian mental health care providers than beneficiaries who use other health care coverage, and that psychiatrists have the lowest acceptance rates of new TRICARE Standard and Extra beneficiaries compared with other providers.[35]

In its 2009 *Access to Mental Health Services* report, DOD noted that two reasons most cited by civilian mental health providers, including psychiatrists, for not accepting new TRICARE patients were "not aware of TRICARE" and "reimbursement." DOD also reported that TMA would increase outreach to mental health providers in selected locations to improve awareness of the program. In addition to the increased outreach, DOD also reported two initiatives designed to enhance beneficiaries' access to mental health care—the Telemental Health Program and the TRICARE Assistance Program. The Telemental Health Program[36] connects TRICARE beneficiaries in one office to civilian mental health providers in another medical office through an audiovisual link. The TRICARE Assistance Program[37] is a Web-based program that enables certain beneficiaries to contact licensed civilian counselors 24 hours a day for short-term, nonmedical issues.[38] Also, in recognition that mental health is an issue of concern for its beneficiaries, each of the TRICARE Regional Offices and contractors has established staff positions that focus specifically on mental health issues, including access to care.

More recently, the NDAA for fiscal year 2010 required DOD to report on the appropriate number of personnel to meet the mental health care needs of servicemembers, retired members, and dependents and to develop and implement a plan to significantly increase the number of DOD military and civilian mental health personnel, among other requirements.[39] In response to this requirement, DOD reported in February 2011 that it has identified criteria for the military services to use in determining the appropriate number of mental health personnel needed to meet the needs of their beneficiaries.[40] However, DOD also noted that the military services are still testing and validating these criteria to determine how effective they would be in gauging adequate mental health staffing numbers. Therefore, although DOD reported increases in the number of mental health providers employed at military treatment facilities or contracted to join TRICARE's network of providers, it did not specifically estimate the appropriate number of mental health care providers needed. DOD also reported that initiatives are under way to increase the number of mental health providers in military treatment facilities, including increasing the number of Public Health Service providers serving in military treatment facilities as well as recruitment and retention incentives. These initiatives, if successfully implemented, could reduce the demand for civilian mental health providers in those locations.

ALTHOUGH TMA HAS TYPICALLY USED FEEDBACK MECHANISMS TO GAUGE TRICARE STANDARD AND EXTRA BENEFICIARIES' ACCESS TO CIVILIAN PROVIDERS, IT IS DEVELOPING A NEW METHOD FOR MONITORING ACCESS

TMA and its contractors have used various feedback mechanisms, such as surveys, to gauge beneficiaries' access to care under TRICARE Standard and Extra. More recently, TMA officials have taken steps to develop a model to help identify geographic areas where beneficiaries that use TRICARE Standard and Extra may experience access problems. However, because this initiative is still evolving, it is too early to determine its effectiveness.

TMA Has Primarily Relied on Feedback Mechanisms to Gauge Beneficiaries' Access to Civilian Providers under TRICARE Standard and Extra

TMA has primarily relied on feedback to gauge beneficiaries' access to civilian providers under TRICARE Standard and Extra, as historically, access to care has only been routinely monitored for beneficiaries enrolled in TRICARE Prime, the only option with access standards.[41] These feedback mechanisms have included surveys of civilian health care (including mental health care) providers as well as surveys of nonenrolled beneficiaries who are eligible to use the TRICARE Standard and Extra options as well as TRICARE Reserve Select. Additionally, TMA and its contractors use feedback from beneficiaries' inquiries and complaints to help identify problems with access, among other issues.

In fiscal year 2005, TMA implemented its first multiyear survey of civilian providers (network and nonnetwork) as required by the NDAA 2004. TMA's survey was supposed to assess beneficiaries' access to civilian providers under the TRICARE Standard and Extra options by determining whether civilian providers would accept these beneficiaries as new patients. In 2006, we reported on TMA's survey methodology, among other issues, and reported that it was sound and statistically valid. TMA's results for this first multiyear survey of civilian providers, which was fielded through 2007, showed that about 8 of 10 physicians and behavioral health providers accepted TRICARE beneficiaries as new patients, if they accepted any patients at all.[42] However, while these results appear favorable, as we reported in 2006, there is no benchmark with which to compare them.

Subsequently, the NDAA 2008 required TMA to conduct two multiyear surveys—one of civilian providers and one of nonenrolled beneficiaries— to determine the adequacy of access to health care and mental health care for these beneficiaries. In March 2010, we reported[43] that the methodology for both of TMA's surveys was sound and generally addressed the methodological requirements outlined in the law.[44] TMA has completed the first 2 years (2008 and 2009) of these surveys.

TMA and its contractors also use feedback collected from beneficiaries' inquiries and complaints to identify and gauge potential problem areas, including issues with access to care. However, this type of feedback is not representative because not every beneficiary who has a question or complaint will contact TMA or its contractors. TMA uses its Assistance Reporting Tool to collect and analyze information on the beneficiary inquiries that it receives, including inquiries on access to care from beneficiaries who use TRICARE Standard and Extra.[45] During fiscal years 2008 through 2010, data from the Assistance Reporting Tool showed that only about 5 percent of closed cases on all TRICARE-related beneficiary inquiries and complaints were from TRICARE Standard and Extra beneficiaries. Further, of the total inquiries and complaints received from these beneficiaries, TMA reported that 313 cases were access-to-care related (2 percent).

The contractors separately receive feedback from beneficiaries through some or all of the following methods: (1) telephone, (2) e-mail, (3) in-person at a TRICARE Service Center, or (4) in writing. Each contractor collects and reports information on their beneficiary feedback differently. In reviewing contractors' data on beneficiary inquiries or complaints received, we found:

- During fiscal year 2009, TMA's contractor in the North region reported receiving 11,176 (less than 1 percent) access-to-care inquiries out of a total of more than 5 million inquiries. This contractor does not categorize its inquiries by TRICARE option, but does collect and categorize inquiries specific to access-to-care concerns. In fiscal year 2010, the contractor received 3,642 access-to-care inquiries (less than 1 percent) out of a total of more than 5 million inquiries.

- TMA's contractor in the South region reported that during calendar year 2009, it received a total of 7,785 complaints. Of these, 175 (2 percent) were submitted by TRICARE Standard and Extra beneficiaries. While access to care did not represent a top reason for their complaints in 2009, this contractor reported that 15 of the complaints received were related to beneficiary appointment and wait times. This contractor also reported that it received a total of 7,927 complaints in calendar year 2010. Of these, 134 (about 2 percent) were submitted by TRICARE Standard and Extra beneficiaries, and only 14 of the 134 complaints were specific to beneficiary appointment and wait times.

- Finally, data submitted to us by TMA's contractor in the West region showed that it received a total of 809 grievances from TRICARE beneficiaries between January 2008 and December 2010. Of these, TRICARE Standard and Extra beneficiaries submitted 83 inquiries (about 10 percent), and about 2 percent of the 83 inquiries were specific to provider appointment wait times.

TMA Has Initiated Steps to Establish a Method for Routinely Monitoring Access to Civilian Providers for TRICARE Standard and Extra Beneficiaries

TMA has recently initiated steps to establish an approach to routinely monitor beneficiaries' access to both network and nonnetwork providers under the TRICARE Standard and Extra options. (The new approach will also apply to beneficiaries using the TRICARE Reserve Select option.) In recognition that the military health system had no established measures for determining the adequacy of network and nonnetwork providers for these beneficiaries, in February 2010, TMA's Office of Policy and Operations directed the TRICARE Regional Offices to develop a model to identify geographic areas where they may experience access problems as well as areas of provider shortages for the general population. The model is intended to help the TRICARE Regional Offices and their contractors identify geographic areas where additional efforts to increase access to civilian providers may be warranted.

To implement this approach, TMA recommended that each regional office adapt and standardize the model that had originally been developed by its West regional office in 2008. This model applies a specific provider-to-beneficiary ratio based on the Graduate Medical Education National Advisory Committee's recommended standards for health care services[46] to different provider specialties to determine whether there are sufficient numbers and types of providers for the nonenrolled beneficiary population in certain locations. To identify locations for analysis, West regional office officials used zip codes to identify locations with populations of 500 or more nonenrolled beneficiaries. According to officials in the West regional office, they then identified the network and nonnetwork providers who practiced and had previously accepted a TRICARE patient in these same locations and applied a specific provider-to-beneficiary ratio against each provider specialty included in the model for the locations assessed. Each regional office has developed a model that generally follows the same methodology and includes similar data as the West regional office's model, although variations exist. For example, while one regional office includes provider data that represents 15 provider specialties, another regional office includes 40 provider specialties in its model. Officials at one regional office told us they have plans to update their model to reflect changes in the beneficiary population, and an official at another regional office said that staff were already in the process of updating their model, which may include additional provider demographic factors.

TMA directed each TRICARE Regional Office to apply the model at least semiannually beginning on May 1, 2010. According to officials in TMA's South region, they plan to apply the model semi-annually as directed while TMA's regional offices in the North and West apply the model as needed. More specifically, since TMA's office in the North region implemented the model, it has assessed 20 locations, and now applies the model as needed in response to specific concerns. Meanwhile, officials from TMA's office in the West region told us that they initially applied the model to over 50 locations and that they now apply the model as needed, such as in response to a specific inquiry about access to care in a particular location. Officials in the North regional office noted that their model's data are used in conjunction with other indicators to assess if further analysis of civilian provider availability is needed. Officials in the West region said that they plan to reach out to providers in the community or use the contractor to help recruit additional providers to the TRICARE network if the model identifies an area that is short of their targeted number of providers in a given specialty.

Based on our review of each regional office's initial approach, we found this methodology to be reasonable. However, because the regional models were recently developed, it is too early to determine their effectiveness. And, while the regional offices provided us with examples of their models, they did not provide documentation of how they applied a provider-tobeneficiary ratio as criteria to determine the adequacy of access in these locations or any documentation of their results, although they told us that they did not identify any access problems.

TMA's Contractors Educate Civilian Providers about TRICARE and Surveys Indicate That Providers Are Generally Aware of the Program

TMA's contractors educate civilian providers about TRICARE program requirements, policies, and procedures. Contractors also conduct outreach to increase providers' awareness of TRICARE, and TMA's provider survey results indicate providers are generally aware of the program. However, providers' awareness of TRICARE does not necessarily signify that they have an accurate understanding of it.

TMA's Contractors Inform Network and Nonnetwork Providers about TRICARE

Under the second generation of TRICARE contracts, TMA's contractors are required to conduct activities to help ensure that providers—both network and nonnetwork—are aware of TRICARE program requirements, policies, and procedures in their respective regions. To accomplish this, the contractors are required to have active provider education programs. In addition, each contractor must submit an annual marketing and education plan to TMA's Communications and Customer Service office that outlines its methods for educating providers based on contractual requirements. All contractors include details in these plans about their efforts to satisfy requirements to distribute regular bulletins and newsletters as well as educate new network providers, such as through orientation sessions or with a Welcome Tool Kit.[47]

The contractors' marketing and education plans also identify provider education efforts that vary across the regions. These efforts vary because contractors have some flexibility in how they achieve outcomes and because the contractors may include additional performance standards in their contracts.[48] Under the second generation of TRICARE contracts, contractors have added performance standards related to provider education. For example, one contractor must visit high-volume network and nonnetwork providers in its region annually, while another contractor must conduct annual seminars for the network and nonnetwork providers in its Prime Service Areas.[49] TMA reported that each contractor had fulfilled its provider education requirements as of December 2010.

All of the contractors also make TRICARE education resources available to providers. Many of these resources are available on the contractors' Web sites and include the *TRICARE Provider Handbook*[50] as well as quick reference charts that include information on provider resources and TRICARE covered benefits and services, among other topics. One contractor hosts electronic seminars on its Web site that allow providers to learn about the TRICARE program at their convenience. Another contractor has developed a reference chart that details the Prime, Standard, and Extra benefit options and has mailed it to both network and nonnetwork providers in its region who have accepted TRICARE beneficiaries as patients.

In addition, all of the contractors have conducted outreach activities to promote or increase providers' awareness of TRICARE. This has included participating in provider events with local, state, or national groups, including physician associations, medical societies, military treatment facilities, and military associations. Contractors told us that while at these events, they answer providers' questions about the program, distribute TRICARE materials, and encourage providers to join the regional TRICARE network. All of the contractors have also participated in events specific to behavioral health care. Contractors said that these events allow them the opportunity to discuss behavioral health issues that may particularly affect military servicemembers and their families, such as suicide and post-traumatic stress disorder, with providers. The contractors also use social media[51] to highlight TRICARE information for providers, including resources and program news and changes. For example, one contractor used its Twitter account to provide a link to information on how to become a network or TRICARE-authorized provider in its region. Additionally, two of the TRICARE Regional Offices as well as two contractors have specifically conducted outreach related to either encouraging network and nonnetwork providers to accept TRICARE beneficiaries as patients or thanking them for doing so. For example, in January 2011, one contractor mailed letters to nonnetwork providers, encouraging them to support TRICARE beneficiaries by joining the network.

Results of TMA's Provider Surveys Indicate a General Awareness of TRICARE, but May Not Necessarily Signify an Accurate Understanding of the Program

Although TMA's provider surveys indicate a general awareness of the program, these results may not signify an accurate understanding of TRICARE. Survey results from TMA's first multiyear survey (2005 through 2007) of civilian providers (network and nonnetwork) indicated that 87 percent of providers on average were aware of TRICARE. TMA's second multiyear survey of civilian providers (network and nonnetwork),[52] which has completed 2 years (2008 and 2009) of its 4-year cycle, similarly asked whether providers were aware of the TRICARE program. Although the results of this survey are not generalizeable,[53] TMA's results show that, of those providers who responded, 87 percent on average were aware of the program.[54]

Although TMA's survey results indicate that providers were generally aware of TRICARE, this does not necessarily mean that providers had an accurate understanding of the program's options and its requirements. For example, representatives of an association representing current and former servicemembers told us that providers do not always understand the differences between the TRICARE Standard and TRICARE Prime options. Similarly, in a November 2008 report, CNA stated that the providers they interviewed were often confused about the differences between TRICARE Standard and TRICARE Prime.[55] One provider, a former president of a local medical society, said many providers are under the misconception that TRICARE Standard is the same as TRICARE Prime and that when providers have had bad experiences with TRICARE Prime, which generally pays network providers less than Medicare, they end up refusing to accept any TRICARE patients because they "don't want to deal with" a health maintenance organization. This lack of understanding is not always easy to remedy. According to the contractors, because many providers have relatively low volumes of TRICARE patients, it can be challenging to encourage them to take advantage of the available TRICARE education resources or to remain current on updates and changes to the program. In 2009, the average percentage of Prime Service Areas civilian providers' and non-Prime Service Areas civilian providers' TRICARE patient population (under any option) was 5.14 percent and 3. 42 percent, respectively.

TMA'S CONTRACTORS EDUCATE BENEFICIARIES ON ALL TRICARE OPTIONS AND PROVIDE INFORMATION ON NETWORK PROVIDERS; NEW CONTRACTS WILL ALSO REQUIRE INFORMATION ABOUT NONNETWORK PROVIDERS

Under the second generation of TRICARE contracts, TMA's contractors have beneficiary education programs that contain information on all of the TRICARE options; contractors also maintain directories of network providers. Under its third generation of contracts, TMA will also require contractors to include information on nonnetwork providers in their directories.

TMA's Contractors Educate Beneficiaries on all TRICARE Options

Under the second generation of TRICARE contracts, TMA's contractors have established beneficiary education programs that contain information on all of the TRICARE options, including Standard and Extra. To meet its beneficiary education requirements, each contractor must submit an annual marketing and education plan to TMA's Communications and Customer Service office that outlines the contractor's methods for educating beneficiaries based on its contractual requirements. For example, the contractor may include details in its marketing and education plan about intentions to distribute required beneficiary newsletters and handbooks, which include information on TRICARE's options and covered services. These plans also specify how the contractors are to provide required weekly one-hour TRICARE briefings to audiences specified by the commanders of their regional military treatment facilities. TMA reported that each of the contractors had fulfilled its beneficiary education requirements as of December 2010.

TMA has only one beneficiary education requirement targeted to TRICARE Standard and Extra beneficiaries: contractors must provide these beneficiaries with the annual *TRICARE Standard Health Matters* newsletter. The 2010 *TRICARE Standard Health Matters* newsletter included articles on topics such as waiving cost-sharing for certain preventive services under TRICARE Standard and Extra. In 2010, the contractors mailed this newsletter to approximately 1.1 million TRICARE Standard and Extra households and made it available electronically through e-mail and their Web sites.[56] Additionally, for the first time, in summer 2010 TMA developed a second *TRICARE Standard Health Matters* newsletter for TRICARE Standard and Extra beneficiaries in an electronic format as an additional resource to fill any possible information gaps to beneficiaries. The contractors then e-mailed the electronic newsletter to beneficiaries and posted it to their Web sites.[57] This electronic newsletter included articles on topics such as how beneficiaries may save money by using TRICARE Extra and how they can stay informed about TRICARE. Two of the contractors told us that it is difficult to communicate with TRICARE Standard and Extra beneficiaries because they do not necessarily have ready access to the beneficiaries' residential or e-mail addresses as these beneficiaries are not required to enroll. This lack of information can make communicating with these beneficiaries challenging, and as a result, TRICARE Standard and Extra beneficiaries may not receive all the available information on their TRICARE benefit. A TMA official noted that TMA is not considering making the additional electronic newsletter a requirement of the third generation of TRICARE contracts, although the contractors may use it to communicate with beneficiaries.

All of the contractors also make additional TRICARE education resources available to beneficiaries. Many of these resources are available on their Web sites, and may include the *TRICARE Standard Handbook*[58] and brochures that explain the different TRICARE options and costs to beneficiaries, among other topics. For example, one contractor makes games available on its Web site, which enables beneficiaries to interactively learn about the TRICARE program. Another contractor posts its own monthly newsletter to its Web site, through which beneficiaries receive information about TRICARE, including its different options, and activities specific to its region. Meanwhile, the third contractor has developed several different fact sheets for beneficiaries that summarize key TRICARE program elements in short, easy-to-read formats.

Each of the three contractors also conducts outreach to enhance beneficiaries' awareness of TRICARE. For example, each of the contractors has attended events hosted by organizations such as the Military Officers Association of America, the Enlisted Association of the National Guard of the United States, the National Military Family Association, the Military Health System, and the Adjutants General Association of the United States. Contractors stated that while at these events they can share TRICARE information with attendees. One contractor also noted that while at these events it addresses beneficiaries' concerns and directs them to further resources. Contractors also use social media to communicate with beneficiaries and provide information on different TRICARE topics, including (1) benefits, (2) resources, and (3) health campaigns. For instance, one contractor used its Facebook page to clarify whether TRICARE Standard beneficiaries needed primary care managers to coordinate their referrals. Another contractor included information on Facebook about how beneficiaries could access information about their TRICARE benefit.

Contractors Provide Directories of Network Providers to Facilitate Access to Care; New Contracts Will Also Require Information on Nonnetwork Providers

To facilitate beneficiaries' access to care, TMA requires its contractors to maintain directories of TRICARE-authorized network providers. These directories are to include current information (updated within 30 days) about each network provider, including specialty, address, and telephone number. The contractors are required to make their directories readily accessible to all beneficiaries, and as a result, all of the contractors' Web sites have online provider directories.

Under the second generation of TRICARE contracts, TMA does not require its contractors to provide similar information on nonnetwork providers. However, beneficiaries may contact the TRICARE Regional Offices or the contractors for assistance in locating a network or nonnetwork provider. Two of the contractors said they currently collect information on nonnetwork providers who have accepted TRICARE beneficiaries and can use this information to assist beneficiaries in locating a nonnetwork provider. Beneficiaries can also use TMA's TRICARE Web site, which refers beneficiaries to the American Medical Association's provider directory and the *Yellow Pages*, to find a nonnetwork provider. However, these online resources do not indicate whether a provider is TRICARE-authorized or has accepted TRICARE patients in the past.

TMA recognized that its Web site asked beneficiaries to "start from square one" to identify a TRICARE-authorized nonnetwork provider. Although it is not a routine practice for insurance companies to identify nonnetwork providers in their online directories, in February 2010, TMA's Deputy Chief of TRICARE Policy and Operations recommended (through a memo) that TMA establish an online search tool on its Web site to enable beneficiaries to identify both network and nonnetwork providers no later than May 1, 2010. However, TMA noted that it did not have sufficient data to develop this online search tool.

Instead, TMA officials decided that under the third generation of TRICARE contracts, each contractor would be responsible for creating an online provider directory for its region that would include information for beneficiaries on TRICARE-authorized providers, both network and nonnetwork.

AGENCY COMMENTS

We received comments on a draft of this report from DOD. DOD concurred with our overall findings and provided technical comments, which we incorporated where appropriate.

Randall B. Williamson
Director, Health Care

APPENDIX I: TRICARE REIMBURSEMENT RATES THAT REMAIN HIGHER THAN MEDICARE REIMBURSEMENT RATES

Beginning in fiscal year 1991, in an effort to control escalating costs, Congress instructed the Department of Defense (DOD) to gradually lower its reimbursement rates for individual civilian providers to mirror those paid by

Medicare.[1] Congress specified that reductions were not to exceed 15 percent in a given year.

As of March 2011, there were seven nonmaternity procedures or services for which reimbursement remains higher under TRICARE than Medicare. (See table 4.)

Table 4. TRICARE Reimbursement Rates That Remain Higher than Medicare Reimbursement Rates for Nonmaternity Procedures and Services

CPT code[a]	Procedure or service performed	Ratio of TRICARE to Medicare reimbursement
36591	Collection of blood specimen from a completely implantable venous access device	1.017
38240	Bone marrow or blood-derived peripheral stem cell transplantation; allogenic	1.152
38241	Bone marrow or blood-derived peripheral stem cell transplantation; autologous	1.155
86901	Blood typing; Rh (D)	1.810
92953	Temporary transcutaneous pacing	1.210
99173	Screening test of visual acuity, quantitative, bilateral	3.466
99359	Prolonged evaluation and management service before and/or after direct (face-to-face) patient care; each additional 30 minutes	1.076

Source: TRICARE Management Activity and the American Medical Association.

[a] Current procedural terminology is a set of codes, descriptions, and guidelines intended to describe procedures and services performed by physicians and other health care providers.

Additionally, beginning in 1998, the TRICARE Management Activity (TMA) established a policy that its reimbursement rates for some maternity services and procedures must be set at the higher of the current Medicare fee or the 1997 Medicare fee.[2]

As a result, the TRICARE reimbursement rates for 36 maternity services and procedures are higher than Medicare. (See table 5.)

Table 5. TRICARE Reimbursement Rates That Remain Higher than Medicare Reimbursement Rates for Maternity Procedures and Services

CPT code[a]	Procedure or service performed	Ratio of TRICARE to Medicare reimbursement
58300	Insertion of intrauterine device	1.038
58600	Ligation or transection of fallopian tube(s), abdominal or vaginal approach, unilateral or bilateral	1.070
58605	Ligation or transection of fallopian tube(s), abdominal or vaginal approach, postpartum, unilateral or bilateral, during same hospitalization (separate procedure)	1.015
58615	Occlusion of fallopian tube(s) by device (e.g., band, clip, Falope ring) vaginal or suprapubic approach	1.118
58970	Follicle puncture for oocyte retrieval, any method	1.004
59012	Cordocentesis (intrauterine), any method	1.200
59020	Fetal contraction stress test	1.327
59025	Fetal non-stress test	1.055
59030	Fetal scalp blood sampling	1.487
59050	Fetal monitoring during labor by consulting physician (e.g., non-attending physician) with written report; supervision and interpretation	1.400
59051	Fetal monitoring during labor by consulting physician (e.g. non-attending physician) with written report; interpretation only	1.285
59135	Surgical treatment of ectopic pregnancy; interstitial, uterine pregnancy requiring total hysterectomy	1.127
59140	Surgical treatment of ectopic pregnancy; cervical, with evacuation	1.093
59160	Curettage, postpartum	1.136
59320	Cerclage of cervix, during pregnancy; vaginal	1.178
59325	Cerclage of cervix, during pregnancy; abdominal	1.296
59350	Hysterorrhaphy of ruptured uterus	1.276
59409	Vaginal delivery only (with or without episiotomy and/or forceps)	1.318
59410	Vaginal delivery only (with or without episiotomy and/or forceps); including postpartum care	1.135
59412	External cephalic version, with or without tocolysis	1.307
59414	Delivery of placenta (separate procedure)	1.397
59514	Cesarean delivery only	1.361
59515	Cesarean delivery only; including postpartum care	1.087
59525	Subtotal or total hysterectomy after cesarean delivery	1.032
59612	Vaginal delivery only, after previous cesarean delivery (with or without episiotomy and/or forceps)	1.239

Table 5. (Continued)

CPT code[a]	Procedure or service performed	Ratio of TRICARE to Medicare reimbursement
59614	Vaginal delivery only, after previous cesarean delivery (with or without episiotomy and/or forceps); including postpartum care	1.093
59620	Cesarean delivery only, following attempted vaginal delivery after previous cesarean delivery	1.373
59622	Cesarean delivery only, following attempted vaginal delivery after previous cesarean delivery; including postpartum care	1.098
59840	Induced abortion, by dilation and curettage	1.237
59850	Induced abortion, by one or more intra-amniotic injections (amniocentesis-injections), including hospital admission and visits, delivery of fetus and secundines	1.160
59851	Induced abortion, by one or more intra-amniotic injections (amniocentesis-injections), including hospital admission and visits, delivery of fetus and secundines; with dilation and curettage and/or evacuation	1.042
59852	Induced abortion, by one or more intra-amniotic injections (amniocentesis-injections), including hospital admission and visits, delivery of fetus and secundines; with hysterectomy (failed intra-amniotic injection)	1.125
59855	Induced abortion, by one or more vaginal suppositories (e.g., prostaglandin) with or without cervical dilation (e.g. laminaria), including hospital admission and visits, delivery of fetus and secundines	1.010
59856	Induced abortion, by one or more vaginal suppositories (e.g., prostaglandin) with or without cervical dilation (e.g. laminaria), including hospital admission and visits, delivery of fetus and secundines; with dilation and curettage and/or evacuation	1.060
59857	Induced abortion, by one or more vaginal suppositories (e.g., prostaglandin) with or without cervical dilation (e.g. laminaria), including hospital admission and visits, delivery of fetus and secundines; with hysterotomy (failed-medical evacuation)	1.229
59866	Multifetal pregnancy reduction(s)	1.365

Source: TRICARE Management Activity and the American Medical Association.

[a] Current procedural terminology is a set of codes, descriptions, and guidelines intended to describe procedures and services performed by physicians and other health care providers.

APPENDIX II: TMA'S STUDIES ON TRICARE REIMBURSEMENT RATES

TMA contracted with a health-policy research and consulting firm to conduct a number of studies about specific TRICARE reimbursement rates. Some of these studies resulted in changes to the TRICARE reimbursement rates for certain procedures. A brief description of these studies is provided below.

Studies of Reimbursement Rates for Specific Maternity/Delivery Procedures, 2006 through 20111

Starting in 2006, TMA's consultant has conducted annual comparisons of TRICARE's reimbursement rates for certain maternity/delivery procedures with Medicaid[2] reimbursement rates on a state-by-state basis. Any reimbursement rates that were found to be below the Medicaid level of payment have been increased.

- For 2006, TMA found that for at least one procedure, the Medicaid rates in 12 states were higher than TRICARE reimbursement rates.[3]
- For 2007, TMA found that for at least one procedure, the Medicaid rates in 11 states were higher than TRICARE reimbursement rates.[4]
- For 2008, TMA found that for at least one procedure, the Medicaid rates in 18 states were higher than TRICARE reimbursement rates.
- For 2009, TMA found that for at least one procedure, the Medicaid rates in 19 states were higher than TRICARE reimbursement rates.
- For 2010, TMA found that for at least one procedure, the Medicaid rates in the same 19 states were higher than TRICARE reimbursement rates.
- For 2011, TMA found that 3 of the 19 states from 2010 no longer met the criteria of having at least one maternity/delivery procedure with TRICARE reimbursement rates lower than Medicaid. As a result, for at least one procedure, the Medicaid rates in 16 states were higher than TRICARE reimbursement rates.

Comparison of Commercial, Medicaid, and TRICARE Reimbursement Rates for Selected Medical Specialties, April 2009[6]

TMA's consultant compared specific TRICARE reimbursement rates with reimbursement rates from Medicaid and commercial insurers. For the comparison with Medicaid rates, it identified commonly used procedures for 13 medical specialties[7] and compared TRICARE's reimbursement rates for these procedures with Medicaid's fee-for-service rates in 49 states.[8] Overall, the median value of the 2009 Medicaid rates in the 49 states was about 18 percent lower than TRICARE's reimbursement rates. In 24 states, the TRICARE reimbursement rates exceeded the state Medicaid program rates for the 13 medical specialties reviewed. Conversely, the study found that in 3 states—New Mexico, Arizona, and Wyoming—Medicaid rates, on average, exceeded the TRICARE reimbursement rates for these 13 specialties. For the comparison with commercial rates, TMA's consultant analyzed reimbursement amounts for 12 medical specialties[9] in 15 geographic market areas[10] and found that commercial rates were higher than TRICARE reimbursement rates for these 12 specialties in almost all of the geographic market areas analyzed.

Review of TRICARE Reimbursement Rates for Pediatric Vaccines and Immunizations, January 2009[11]

TMA's consultant studied TRICARE's reimbursement rates for selected pediatric immunizations and vaccines to determine whether TRICARE's reimbursement amounts were below the cost that pediatricians must pay to acquire these vaccines.[12] It analyzed 15 vaccines codes (which often have more than one type of vaccine product associated with them) and found that for each of the vaccine codes, TRICARE's reimbursement rates exceeded the average acquisition cost paid by pediatric providers for at least one of the vaccine products. Overall, in 2007 TRICARE's reimbursement rates exceeded the average acquisition cost for the 15 vaccine codes by 30 percent (when weighted by volume). The study also noted that some pediatricians may pay more than the average acquisition price, and some network pediatricians may receive TRICARE reimbursement rates below the average acquisition cost if they have agreed to reimbursement discounts as a condition of belonging to the TRICARE provider network.[13] The study also compared TRICARE's reimbursement rates to those of Medicare and Medicaid. The study noted that

TRICARE uses the same vaccine prices and administration prices as Medicare for vaccine codes for which Medicare sets a price (which is mostly at 106 percent of the average sales price of the vaccine as of 2005— determined by the Centers for Medicare & Medicaid Services). For those vaccines for which Medicare does not have a set price, TRICARE reimbursement rates are set at 95 percent of average wholesale price— which is essentially a "list price" set by the manufacturer. When compared to Medicaid's rates, TRICARE's reimbursement rate for the administration of a vaccine or immunization was higher than Medicaid's in every state in 2008.[14]

Analysis of TRICARE Payment Rates for Maternity/Delivery Services, Evaluation and Management Services, and Pediatric Immunizations, March 2006[15]

TMA's consultant compared TRICARE's reimbursement rates for 14 specific maternity/delivery services and a pediatrician office visit[16] with Medicaid[17] and commercial payment rates.[18] It found the following:

- For these specific maternity/delivery services, TRICARE's reimbursement rates were higher than Medicaid rates in 35 of the 45 states reviewed. Additionally, in 27 of the 35 states, the Medicaid payment rate for deliveries was less than 90 percent of TRICARE's reimbursement rates. TRICARE's reimbursement rates for deliveries were less than the median commercial rates in all but one of the 50 markets studied (they were equivalent in the remaining market). Overall, the median commercial rates for deliveries were 24 percent higher than TRICARE's reimbursement rates in 2005.
- For pediatric care, TRICARE's reimbursement rate for a mid-level office visit for an established patient (the most commonly billed code by pediatricians) was higher than the state Medicaid reimbursement rate in 41 of the 45 states in 2005.[19] However, the median commercial reimbursement rates were 10 percent higher than TRICARE's reimbursement rates in the 50 TRICARE markets examined.
- TRICARE's reimbursement for pediatric vaccines and injectable drugs generally appeared to be reasonable when derived from Medicare pricing, based on an analysis of private sector costs, average wholesale prices, and average sales prices for top volume CPT codes. However, TRICARE's reimbursement rate for the pediatric and

adolescent dose of the hepatitis A vaccine was found to be 22 percent lower than estimated private sector costs to obtain the vaccine in 2005. Specifically, the TRICARE reimbursement rate for this vaccine dose was $22.64, while pediatricians were paying between $27.41 and $30.37 for the vaccine. Based on the results of this study, TMA used its general authority to deviate from Medicare rates (upon which TRICARE rates are based),[20] and starting May 1, 2006, TMA instructed the contractors to reimburse pediatric hepatitis A vaccines nationally at a new reimbursement rate of $30.40.

APPENDIX III: TMA'S USE OF WAIVERS

TMA has the authority to increase TRICARE reimbursement rates for network and nonnetwork civilian providers to ensure that all beneficiaries, including TRICARE Standard and Extra beneficiaries, have adequate access to civilian providers. TMA's authorities include: (1) issuing locality waivers that increase rates for specific procedures in specific localities,[1] (2) issuing network waivers that increase some network civilian providers' reimbursements,[2] and (3) restoring TRICARE reimbursement rates in specific localities to the levels that existed before a reduction was made to align TRICARE reimbursement rates with Medicare rates for both network and nonnetwork providers.[3]

Locality waivers may be used to increase rates for specific medical services in specific areas where access to civilian providers has been severely impaired. The resulting rate increase would be applied to both network and nonnetwork civilian providers for the medical services identified in the areas where access is impaired. A total of 17 applications for locality waivers have been submitted to TMA between January 2002 and January 2011. TMA approved 16 of these waivers. (See table 6.)

Table 6. Applications for Locality Waivers and Approval Results

Date submitted	Affected location	Affected services	Amount of increase requested	Outcome
1/23/03	Juneau, Alaska	All gynecological procedures or services delivered by one provider	600 percent[a]	3/26/03— Approved for nonroutine gynecological procedures or services

Date submitted	Affected location	Affected services	Amount of increase requested	Outcome
8/01/04	Fairbanks, Alaska	All inpatient internal medicine procedures or services delivered by providers employed by Fairbanks Memorial Hospital	Veterans Affairs rates	10/28/04— Approved
6/08/05	Anchorage, Alaska	All medical procedures or services delivered by perinatologists	40 percent	11/21/05— Approved for perinatologists who are participating providers[b] 11/21/07— Decreased the rate to 35 percent as a result of an increase in overall TRICARE reimbursement rates in Alaska
6/08/05	Fairbanks, Alaska	Four medical procedures or services delivered by two plastic surgeons	Veterans Affairs rates	5/18/06— Approved to increase rates to the rate paid by the Veterans Affairs for professional services provided by plastic surgeons in Alaska
3/03/05	Puerto Rico[c]	All medical procedures or services delivered by neurosurgeons	40 percent	10/26/05— Approved
Annual study[d] (originally requested on 10/19/05)	Multiple states[e]	14 obstetrical procedures or services	Medicaid reimbursement amounts	3/01/10— Approved
2/23/06	Fairbanks, Alaska	All anesthesia or pain management and treatment services delivered by anesthesiologists	200 percent	6/02/06— Approved to increase rates by 252 percent[f]

Table 6. (Continued)

Date submitted	Affected location	Affected services	Amount of increase requested	Outcome
7/17/06[g]	Puerto Ricoc	Medical procedures or services delivered by perinatologists, orthopedists, and pediatric urologists	Various: 310 percent for perinatologists; 300 percent for orthopedists; and 162 percent for pediatric urologists	Denied because the request did not meet the requirements for a locality waiver
7/01/06[g]	All of Alaska	All medical procedures or services	Veterans Affairs rates	1/01/07— Approved
8/07/06[g]	Fairbanks, Alaska	Three services delivered by a pulmonologist	Veterans Affairs rates	12/13/06— Approved
5/24/07[g]	Juneau, Alaska	All orthopedic and physical medicine rehabilitation at Juneau Bone & Joint Center	15 percent	8/06/07— Approved
12/18/07[g]	Key West, Florida	All psychiatric services in the code range of 90800 through 90899 delivered by two providers	50 percent	1/07/08— Approved for patients 18 and under within the 33040 zip code
4/16/08[g]	Puerto Ricoc	All medically indicated bilateral breast reduction surgeries delivered by surgeons	$2,600 (bilateral procedure)	6/19/08— Approved
8/22/08[g]	Juneau, Alaska	Orthopedic and physical medicine/rehabilitation services at Juneau Bone & Joint Center	35 percent	9/05/08— Approved
5/05/09g	Anchorage/ Palmer, Alaska	Neurosurgical services for three provider groups	250 percent	7/14/09— Approved
8/20/09[g]	Anchorage area, Alaska	Pain management services for four provider groups in and around the Anchorage area	217 percent	11/17/09— Approved
11/13/09[g]	All of Alaska	Certain rheumatology, orthopedics, and	Various: 125 percent for	12/30/09— Approved for

Date submitted	Affected location	Affected services	Amount of increase requested	Outcome
		otolaryngology services	rheumatologists; between 150 and 175 percent for orthopedists; and 175 percent for otolaryngologists	certain rheumatology, orthopedics, and otolaryngology services provided by the 14 practices which have signed letters of intent to provide these services, as well as any other practices which sign a letter of intent to provide these services

Source: GAO analysis of TRICARE Management Activity (TMA) data.

[a] Request did not include a specific increase amount. The approved waiver was for the lesser of billed charges or 600 percent of the TRICARE reimbursement rate.

[b] Participating providers submit claims for reimbursement and accept the TRICARE reimbursement rate as payment in full.

[c] The TRICARE Regional Offices are not responsible for managing TRICARE in Puerto Rico because it operates under a different contract than what is used for the three TRICARE regions.

[d] When reviewing the need for this rate adjustment, TMA annually compares TRICARE reimbursement rates with Medicaid rates in states for which data are available. The 19 states listed were identified as needing a rate adjustment based on this analysis. The first of these waivers was approved in 2006 and included only 12 states. Each year when the TRICARE reimbursement rates are adjusted, TMA intends to similarly determine where this adjustment is needed.

[e] The states are Alabama, Arizona, Connecticut, Georgia, Massachusetts, Montana, Nebraska, New Mexico, New York, North Dakota, Oregon, Pennsylvania, South Carolina, South Dakota, Vermont, Virginia, Washington, West Virginia, and Wyoming.

[f] Because the TRICARE reimbursement rate changed during the period between the application and the approval of this waiver, TMA raised the percentage of the increase.

[g] According to TMA, these dates are the dates the waiver submission was assigned or received by TMA to better reflect when TMA started to take action on the request.

Table 7. Applications for Network Waivers and Approval Results

Date submitted	Affected location	Affected services	Amount of increase requested	Outcome
1/29/02	Fredericksburg, Virginia	33 varied medical procedures or services, encompassing various specialties	28 percent[a]	Denied—Application did not substantiate an access-to-care problem
3/07/02	Great Falls, Montana	All medical procedures or services delivered by a specific clinic representing 32 specialties	200 percent[a]	Denied—Application did not directly request a network waiver and increase could be handled under TRICARE Prime Remote[b]
8/13/02	Idaho	All medical procedures and services	15 percent	1/15/03—Approved for nine specialties in the Mountain Home Air Force Base Prime Service Area
12/20/02	Bozeman, Montana	All obstetrical or gynecological medical procedures or services	15 percent	Denied—Increase available under TRICARE Prime Remote[b]
4/08/03	Cheyenne, Wyoming	Three newborn inpatient medical procedures or services	To match civilian insurers' rates	7/16/03—Approved increase to 15 percent above TRICARE reimbursement rates
2/03 and 3/03	Watertown, New York, Norwich, Connecticut	Deliveries provided by nurse midwives in New York and emergency gynecological services in Connecticut	Not specified	Denied–Incomplete application package submitted
9/26/03	Ft. Leonard Wood and Springfield, Missouri	All medical procedures and services delivered by network providers	15 percent	12/24/03—Approved for 11 specialties in Ft. Leonard Wood

Date submitted	Affected location	Affected services	Amount of increase requested	Outcome
				Prime Service Area. Denied for Springfield
1/05/05	Delta Junction and Tok, Alaska	All primary care medical procedures and services	15 percent	3/30/05— Approved for nonmental health medical care services, excluding laboratory services
6/10/05	Norfolk, Virginia	All medical procedures and services for three specialties delivered by a group of pediatric specialists	15 percent	7/08/05— Approved
3/06/06	Rapid City, South Dakota	All obstetrical or gynecological services delivered by a group of specialists	Not specified	5/16/2006— Approved a 15 percent increase for one group of obstetricians and gynecologists
2/16/07[c]	Ellsworth Air Force Base, South Dakota	Evaluation and management codes for orthopedic and rheumatology services by the Black Hills Orthopedic and Spine Center	15 percent	7/13/07— Approved
2/26/07[c]	Fort Bliss, Texas	Opthalmology services provided by Southwest Retina Consultants	15 percent	Denied because the documentation was not sufficient to support and justify the waiver
1/04/10[c]	Hawaii	Inpatient neonatal and pediatric services by providers at Kapiolani Medical Specialists	15 percent	2/25/10— Approved

Source: GAO analysis of TRICARE Management Activity (TMA) data.

[a] According to TMA, the waiver requesters did not understand that the maximum network waiver is 15 percent over TRICARE reimbursement rates. If the waiver had been granted it would have been limited to 115 percent of the TRICARE reimbursement rate.

ᵇTRICARE Prime Remote is a specialized version of TRICARE Prime available for active duty members when they are assigned to duty stations in areas not served by the military health care system. Under this program, civilian network providers can be reimbursed up to 15 percent above the TRICARE reimbursement rate. Family members who reside with servicemembers who are enrolled in TRICARE Prime Remote are eligible to enroll in and receive care under TRICARE Prime Remote for Active Duty Family Members.
ᶜ According to TMA, these dates are the dates the waiver submission was assigned or received by TMA to better reflect when TMA started to take action on the request.

TMA can also use its authority to restore TRICARE reimbursement rates in specific localities to the levels that existed before a reduction was made to align TRICARE rates with Medicare rates. On two occasions previously, TMA has used this authority in Alaska to encourage both network and nonnetwork civilian providers to accept TRICARE beneficiaries as patients in an effort to ensure adequate access to care. In 2000, TMA used this waiver authority to uniformly increase reimbursement rates for network and nonnetwork civilian providers in rural Alaska, and in 2002, TMA implemented this same waiver for network and nonnetwork civilian providers in Anchorage. However, in 2007 TMA implemented a demonstration project in Alaska that increased reimbursement rates to match those of the Department of Veterans Affairs. As a result, the waivers implemented under this authority were ended. As of January 2011, TMA did not have any waivers of reimbursement rate reductions in place.

APPENDIX IV: ACCESS-TO-CARE CONCERNS IN ALASKA

Access to health care in Alaska is hindered by unique impediments due to its geographically remote location and small population base, which has resulted in some of the highest costs for providing services in the country. To identify and examine the unique access concerns for Alaska, we reviewed the *Interagency Access to Health Care in Alaska Task Force Report to Congress*. We also spoke with TMA officials and a representative of the Alaska State Medical Association to obtain their views on the unique access challenges in this state.

Federal health programs[1] are the leading payer of health care services to Alaska citizens, constituting approximately 31 percent of total health care expenditures in the state in 2006.[2] In 2010, the Department of Health and

Human Services reported that about 14 percent of the population in Alaska had received health care from either DOD's TRICARE program or from the Veterans Health Administration.[3] According to a 2009 study by the Alaska Center for Rural Health, Alaska has a shortage of providers that has been further impacted by its remoteness, harsh climate, and scarce training resources.[4] Workforce shortages in urban areas range from a complete lack of certain specialists in Fairbanks and other towns, to a relative shortage of primary care providers and many specialists in Anchorage. Moreover, rural areas have far more difficulty attracting qualified candidates than more heavily populated areas, such as Anchorage or Fairbanks. TRICARE officials have identified this overall shortage of providers and providers' reluctance to accept TRICARE reimbursement rates as the main impediments to TRICARE beneficiaries' access to civilian providers in Alaska—regardless of which option they use.

Alaska is part of TRICARE's West region, and until recently, Alaska was the only state for which TMA administered and managed TRICARE directly as well as being the only state that did not have Prime Service Areas with networks of civilian providers.[5] In a November 2010 *Federal Register* notice, DOD announced that the responsibility for administering and managing TRICARE in Alaska would transfer from TMA to the contractor for the West region.[6] Additionally, the notice required the contractor to develop networks of civilian providers in two Prime Service Areas to be established around the military treatment facilities located at Fort Wainwright and Eielson Air Force Base, near Fairbanks, Alaska.

This transition of responsibility took place in January 2011, and TMA expects these Prime Service Areas to be developed by July 2011. Additionally, the West region contractor noted that it expects to receive authorization to develop a third Prime Service Area around Elmendorf Air Force Base in Anchorage in late summer 2011.

TMA has taken actions to address TRICARE beneficiaries' access to civilian providers in Alaska by (1) increasing TRICARE's reimbursement rates through the use of waivers and a demonstration project and (2) participating in a federal task force on the delivery of health care in Alaska. Specifically, in areas where access is impaired, TMA has increased reimbursement rates to encourage civilian providers to accept TRICARE beneficiaries through TMA's reimbursement waivers. Of the 24 waivers in place as of January 2011, 13 are for locations in Alaska.

In addition, TMA began a demonstration project in Alaska in February 2007—originally expected to end in December 2009—that raised reimbursement rates for physicians and other noninstitutional professional providers so that on average, they matched those of the Department of Veterans Affairs. Specifically, TRICARE's 2007 reimbursement rates were increased approximately 35 percent.[7]

In July 2009, TMA conducted a preliminary assessment of the demonstration project and found mixed results. Specifically, TMA's analysis determined that three of seven measures of access to care indicated that access had improved since the beginning of the project, while the other four measures did not show an improvement in access.[8]

Despite this inconclusive assessment, TMA officials in the West region said that the demonstration project and the use of waivers have increased access to care, as the number of providers accepting TRICARE's reimbursement rates increased.

According to these officials, the number of providers that have accepted TRICARE's reimbursement rate went from under 300 before the demonstration project to almost 800, as of July 2010. Although DOD has recognized that there have been mixed results on the effectiveness of the demonstration project, it extended the demonstration project through December 31, 2012.

Finally, in recognition that Alaska has unique health care challenges, Congress established the Interagency Access to Care in Alaska Task Force to review how federal agencies with responsibility for health care services in Alaska are meeting the needs of Alaskans.[9]

The Task Force consisted of members from the following: DOD (including TMA), the Department of Veterans Affairs and its Veterans Health Administration, the Department of Health and Human Services and its Centers for Medicare & Medicaid Services and Indian Health Service, and the U.S. Coast Guard.

In September 2010, the Task Force issued its report recommending that, among other things, federal agencies providing health care reimbursement in Alaska should support current projects to develop a budget-neutral, uniform provider reimbursement rate for similar services for Medicare, TRICARE, and the Veterans Health Administration.[10]

According to TMA officials, TMA is currently reviewing the Task Force's recommendations to develop options within the framework of current law and regulations.

However, the full implementation of the recommendations will be under the direction of the Secretary of Health and Human Services.

APPENDIX V: NETWORK ADEQUACY REPORTING REQUIREMENT OF CONTRACTORS UNDER THE SECOND GENERATION OF TRICARE CONTRACTS

Under the second generation of contracts, TMA's contractors have been required to develop and maintain adequate networks of providers, which are to meet the needs of all TRICARE beneficiaries within Prime Service Areas.[1] In doing so, each contractor uses a different methodology for determining the number of providers needed. Contractors are also required to develop their own systems to continuously monitor and evaluate network adequacy and to submit routine reports to TMA on the status of their provider networks in accordance with contract requirements. Specifically, TMA requires its contractors to submit monthly and quarterly reports on network inadequacy and network adequacy, respectively, and to submit corrective action plans for each instance of network inadequacy.

- The monthly report on network inadequacy must include information on each instance in which a beneficiary enrolled in TRICARE Prime is being referred to: (1) a provider outside of TMA's time or distance standards[2] or (2) a nonnetwork provider. According to TMA officials, network inadequacies may occur because of provider shortages; in such instances, contractors are not held accountable for not meeting access standards. However, other network inadequacies, particularly referrals to nonnetwork providers, may also be due to other factors, such as network providers not accepting new patients or beneficiaries' not wanting to wait for available appointments with network providers who are unable to provide an appointment within TMA's access standards. According to a TMA official, none of the contractors have been cited for not meeting TMA's time and distance standards or for referrals to nonnetwork providers under the second generation of TRICARE contracts.
- Contractors' quarterly reports include: (1) the total number of network providers by specialty, (2) the number of additions and deletions to the network by specialty, and (3) actions to contract with additional providers in areas lacking networks to meet access standards, among other things.

End Notes

[1] Eligible beneficiaries include active duty personnel and their dependents, medically eligible Reserve and National Guard personnel and their dependents, and retirees and their dependents and survivors.

[2] The TRICARE program also offers other options, including TRICARE Reserve Select and TRICARE for Life. TRICARE Reserve Select is a premium-based health plan that qualified Reserve and National Guard members may purchase, with care options that are similar to those of TRICARE Standard and Extra. TRICARE beneficiaries who are eligible for Medicare and enroll in Part B are eligible to receive care under TRICARE for Life.

[3] Eligible beneficiaries may choose not to use TRICARE if, for example, they are covered by another health care plan.

[4] Prime Service Areas are geographic areas determined by the Assistant Secretary of Defense for Health Affairs and are defined by a set of 5-digit zip codes, usually within an approximate 40-mile radius of a military inpatient treatment facility. The managed care support contracts also require the contractors to develop civilian provider networks at all Base Realignment and Closure (BRAC) sites, which are military installations that have been closed or realigned as a result of decisions made by the Commission on Base Realignment and Closure.

[5] A network provider is a provider who has a contractual relationship with the TRICARE regional contractors to provide care at a negotiated rate.

[6] See Pub. L. No. 108-136, § 723, 117 Stat. 1392, 1532-34 (2003) and S. Rep. No. 108-46, at 330 (2003).

[7] GAO, Defense Health Care: Access to Care for Beneficiaries Who Have Not Enrolled in TRICARE's Managed Care Option. GAO-07-48 (Washington, D.C.: Dec. 22, 2006).

[8] See Pub. L. No. 110-181, § 711(a), 122 Stat. 3, 190-91.

[9] GAO, Defense Health Care: 2008 Access to Care Surveys Indicate Some Problems, but Beneficiary Satisfaction Is Similar to Other Health Plans, GAO-10-402 (Washington, D.C.; Mar. 31, 2010).

[10] Department of Defense, Task Force on Mental Health, An Achievable Vision: Report of the Department of Defense Task Force on Mental Health (Falls Church, Va., June 2007).

[11] CNA is a nonprofit research organization that operates the Center for Naval Analyses and the Institute for Public Research.

[12] The contracts included in our review are the second generation of TRICARE contracts. The implementation period for these contracts was set to end on March 31, 2010, with the third generation of contracts to begin implementation on April 1, 2010. However, this timeline was delayed due to bid protests on two of the three contracts.

[13] The TRICARE Prime option has five access-to-care standards that address the following: (1) travel time, (2) appointment wait time, (3) availability and accessibility of emergency services, (4) composition of network specialists, and (5) office wait time. See 32 C.F.R. § 199.17(p)(5) (2010).

[14] TRICARE beneficiaries who choose to receive medical care from providers who are not TRICARE-authorized are responsible for all billed charges. Civilian providers consist of primary care physicians, specialists, certified clinical social workers, certified psychiatric nurse specialists, clinical psychologists, certified marriage and family therapists, pastoral counselors, mental health counselors, and psychiatrists.

[15] Network providers also undergo a formal credentialing process through the contractor. Credentialing includes a review of the provider's training, educational degrees, licensure, practice history, etc.

[16] Beginning in fiscal year 1991, in an effort to control escalating health care costs, Congress instructed DOD to gradually lower its reimbursement rates for individual civilian providers to mirror those paid by Medicare. Congress specified that reductions were not to exceed 15 percent in a given year. See 10 U.S.C. §§ 1079(h), 1086(f).

[17] For example, network providers may determine that only a set amount of their practice— such as 10 or 20 percent—will be allocated to TRICARE patients. When this percentage is met, providers may decline to accept any new TRICARE patients.

[18] Claims analyzed were for services provided in an office or other setting outside of an institution. Claims for services rendered at hospitals, military treatment facilities, and other institutions were excluded. TRICARE for Life claims were excluded as well as claims for medical supplies and from chiropractors and pharmacies.

[19] See GAO-07-48.

[20] TMA's first multiyear survey of civilian providers had approximately 18,000, 18,900, and 19,000 responses in 2005, 2006, and 2007 respectively, for an eligible physician response rate of about 50 percent each year.

[21] The first 2 years of TMA's second multiyear survey of civilian providers had 19,309 responses in 2008 and 19,812 responses in 2009 for a 2-year adjusted response rate of 39 percent. TRICARE's reimbursement rates, along with a lack of awareness of the TRICARE program were tied for the most-cited reasons by providers who were accepting new Medicare patients, but would not accept new TRICARE patients over all regions surveyed.

[22] Levy, Robert A., and Gabay, Mary, Some Additional Findings Related to the Acceptance by Civilian Providers of TRICARE Standard, CNA Research Memorandum D0019101.A2/Final (November 2008). TMA tasked CNA to examine the current participation of civilian providers in the TRICARE program, focusing on potential reasons that may inhibit many of these providers from accepting TRICARE Standard and Extra beneficiaries as patients.

[23] Beginning in fiscal year 1991, in an effort to control escalating health care costs, Congress instructed DOD to gradually lower its reimbursement rates for individual civilian providers to mirror those paid by Medicare. Congress specified that reductions were not to exceed 15 percent in a given year. See 10 U.S.C. §§ 1079(h), 1086(f). As of March 2011, the transition to Medicare rates was nearly complete, and reimbursement rates for only 43 services remain higher than Medicare reimbursement rates. (See app. I for a list of these services.)

[24] The Medicare physician fee schedule is updated annually by the sustainable growth rate system, with the intent of limiting the total growth in Medicare spending for physician services over time. Because of rapid growth in Medicare spending for physician services, the sustainable growth rate has called for fee reductions since 2002. However, congressional action has temporarily averted such fee reductions for 2003 through 2011. Although under current law, Medicare's fees to physicians are scheduled to be reduced by about 29.5 percent in 2012, Congress has considered ways to repeal or replace the sustainable growth rate system for a number of years. See 42 U.S.C. § 1395w-4(d).

[25] For more information on TMA's changes to its physician payment rates for obstetric care, see GAO, TRICARE: Changes to Access Policies and Payment Rates for Services Provided by Civilian Obstetricians, GAO-07-941R (Washington, D.C.: July 31, 2007).

[26] 32 C.F.R. § 199.14(j)(1)(iv)(D) (2010). According to a TMA official, TMA usually defines a locality using one or more zip codes.

27 32 C.F.R. § 199.14(j)(1)(iv)(E) (2010).

28 32 C.F.R. § 199.14(j)(1)(iv)(C) (2010).

29 According to TMA, from fiscal year 2006 to 2009, 44,000 additional civilian providers (network and nonnetwork) accepted TRICARE (a more than 13 percent increase).

30 See for example: Institute of Medicine, Hospital-Based Emergency Care: At the Breaking Point, (Washington, D.C.: The National Academies Press, 2006), and Center for Workforce Studies, Association of American Medical Colleges, Recent Studies and Reports on Physician Shortages in the U.S. (November 2010).

31 TMA has the authority to implement bonus payment programs for physicians in areas determined to be medically underserved areas by the Department of Health and Human Services for Medicare purposes. TMA is generally required to make the bonus payments in the same amounts as authorized for Medicare. See 32 C.F.R. § 199.14(j)(2) (2010).

32 See 42 U.S.C. § 1395l(m). Health Professional Shortage Areas include both urban and rural areas. For example, Fulton County, Georgia, (which could be considered an urban area) contains 90 Health Professional Shortage Areas because it lacks primary and mental health care providers. Likewise, the state of Alaska (which is predominantly considered to be a rural area) contains 141 Health Professional Shortage Areas that lack primary and mental health care providers.

33 American Psychological Association, Presidential Task Force on Military Deployment Services for Youth, Families and Service Members, The Psychological Needs of U.S. Military Service Members and Their Families: A Preliminary Report (Feb. 18, 2007).

34 Department of Defense, Report to Congress: Access to Mental Health Services (Sept. 9, 2009).

35 According to the first 2 years of TMA's second round of provider surveys, less than 46 percent of responding psychiatrists who were accepting any new patients would accept new nonenrolled beneficiaries, compared to almost 69 percent of responding primary care providers and almost 72 percent of responding specialist providers.

36 TMA's Telemental Health Program, which began on August 1, 2009, uses medically supervised, secure audio-visual conferencing to link beneficiaries in one location with mental health care providers in another. These providers can evaluate, treat, and refer patients as necessary by video.

37 TMA's TRICARE Assistance Program, which began on August 1, 2009, allows eligible beneficiaries to access licensed counselors for nonmedical issues including stress management and deployment issues.

38 These beneficiaries include active duty family members and those using TRICARE Reserve Select.

39 The law also required the Secretary of Defense to assess the feasibility of establishing one or more military mental health specialties for officers or enlisted servicemembers and required the secretary of each military department to increase the authorized number of active-duty mental health personnel by at least 25 percent. See Pub. L. No. 111-84, § 714, 123 Stat. 2190, 2381-82 (2009).

40 DOD, Mental Health Personnel Required to Meet Mental Health Care Needs of Service Members, Retired Members, and Dependents; Report to Congress (Feb. 1, 2011).

41 Contractors have only been required to monitor access to care for TRICARE Prime beneficiaries. To do this, contractors are to determine the adequacy of civilian provider networks. Although TRICARE Prime is the only option with required access-to-care standards, network adequacy may also affect nonenrolled beneficiaries who use network providers. (See app. V for information on network adequacy requirements which are used to gauge access to care.)

[42] TMA's reported results showed that on average, 92 percent of civilian providers were accepting any new patients.

[43] See GAO-10-402.

[44] The law also directed DOD to give high priority to locations having high concentrations of Selected Reserve servicemembers, which would likely result in surveying beneficiaries who may be under the TRICARE Reserve Select option. However, TMA did not give a high priority to locations with high concentrations of Selected Reserve members. Instead, for both of its surveys, TMA randomly selected areas to produce results that can be generalized to the populations from which the survey samples were drawn. TMA plans to cover the entire United States at the end of the 4-year survey period, which will include any locations with higher concentrations of Selected Reserve servicemembers.

[45] The Assistance Reporting Tool does not include information reported to the contractors. Implemented in 2001, this tool is used by customer service staff in TRICARE program offices, military treatment facilities, and the uniformed services.

[46] The Graduate Medical Education National Advisory Committee projected the need for and supply of physicians and other providers and developed guidelines for the geographic distribution of physicians.

[47] Welcome Tool Kits are distributed to new providers who join the contractor's developed network, and may include reference charts, the TRICARE Provider Handbook, and a welcome letter.

[48] The second generation of managed care support contracts are performance-based contracts. A performance-based contract includes certain performance standards that those offerors submitting bids must achieve if selected for the contract or they may be subject to certain penalties. In their bids for the contract, offerors may also submit additional performance standards for incorporation into the contract where the request for proposal does not have a minimum standard. Under these managed care support contracts, contractors have different requirements related to provider education due to contractors' submission of additional performance standards during the solicitation period.

[49] While these examples are unique to these contractors' contracts, all three contractors may offer these resources to the providers in their regions.

[50] TMA developed the TRICARE Provider Handbook and updates it annually to inform providers about basic and important information about TRICARE and emphasize key operational aspects of the program and program options. The handbook assists providers in coordinating care for TRICARE beneficiaries, and contains information about specific TRICARE programs, policies, and procedures. Any TRICARE program changes and updates may be communicated periodically through the TRICARE Provider News publications.

[51] Social media refers to services that enable individuals to publicly create, share, and discuss information. These services include Facebook and Twitter.

[52] TMA's second civilian provider survey (2008 and 2009) was fielded as two versions. The first version was fielded to physicians, including psychiatrists. The second version was fielded to nonphysician mental health providers, including: (1) certified marriage and family therapists, (2) mental health counselors, (3) pastoral counselors, (4) certified psychiatric nurse specialists, (5) clinical psychologists, and (6) certified clinical social workers.

[53] TMA's consultant conducted analyses of the responses to determine whether they could be generalized to the populations surveyed and found that their responses could not be generalized. As each survey year's results are cumulative, the results may be generalizable at the end of the 4-year survey period.

[54] The result reported above is from responses to the physician survey.

[55] Levy, Robert A., and Gabay, Mary, Some Additional Findings Related to the Acceptance by Civilian Providers of TRICARE Standard (Nov. 2008, p. 4, 29-30).

[56] TMA's Communications and Customer Service annually provides the contractors with a mail file that includes the residential addresses of TRICARE Standard beneficiaries for the purpose of mailing the annual newsletter. TRICARE Extra beneficiaries are included in this list because they are the same as TRICARE Standard beneficiaries except that they choose to obtain health care from network providers.

[57] Although TRICARE Standard and Extra beneficiaries are not required to enroll, these beneficiaries can sign-up for e-mail alerts that deliver the latest TRICARE information. According to a TMA official, the contractors may also collect beneficiaries' e-mail addresses and use these e-mail addresses to communicate with beneficiaries.

[58] The TRICARE Standard Handbook has been developed to guide TRICARE beneficiaries in using the Standard and Extra options. It explains the different types of TRICARE providers and outlines services covered under TRICARE Standard and Extra as well as costs and requirements.

End Notes for Appendix I

[1] See 10 U.S.C. §§ 1079(h), 1086(f).

[2] According to a TMA official, this TRICARE policy was established in 1998 because Medicare decreased the maternity rates by 10 percent that year. The official also noted that TMA determined this 10 percent decrease would jeopardize access and decided that the rates should not fall below the 1997 levels.

End Notes for Appendix II

[1] See the 2011 report at Kennell, D., Witsberger, C., Doukeris, C., Information on Maternity CMACs for 2011 (Task Order No. 3005-001), Kennell and Associates, Inc. (Feb. 1, 2011). This report contains summaries of all previous analyses beginning in 2006.

[2] Medicaid is the joint federal-state program that provides health care coverage for certain low-income individuals.

[3] TMA's consultant reviewed data from 47 states (all except Tennessee, Delaware, and Rhode Island). A state was identified as having TRICARE reimbursement rates below Medicaid if the TRICARE reimbursement rate in any locality was below the Medicaid rate for any of 6 specific maternity/delivery current procedural terminology (CPT) codes. For any state where at least 1 of these 6 TRICARE reimbursement rates were below the Medicaid rate, the rates for 14 CPT codes (the 6 specific codes plus 8 others) were set at the greater of the TRICARE reimbursement rate or the Medicaid rate.

[4] TMA's consultant reviewed data from the 12 states identified in 2006, as well as Idaho, Oklahoma, Virginia, North Carolina, Maryland, Alabama, Vermont, Utah, Kentucky, New Hampshire, and Illinois.

[5] For the 2008, 2009, 2010, and 2011 studies, TMA's consultant reviewed data from all states except Tennessee.

[6] Kennell, D., Brooks, A., Witsberger, C., Cottrell, L., Caney, K., Comparison of Commercial, Medicaid, and TRICARE Reimbursement Rates for Physicians (Task Order 1005-009), Kennell and Associates, Inc. (Apr. 22, 2009).

[7] In order to capture differences between different types of physicians, TMA's consultant examined 13 specialties that provide the vast majority of physician services to TRICARE beneficiaries. The 13 specialties were (1) general and family practice providers, (2) pediatricians, (3) internists, (4) obstetricians/gynecologists, (5) psychiatrists, (6) psychologists, (7) cardiologists, (8) orthopedic surgeons, (9) radiologists, (10) general surgeons, (11) gastroenterologists, (12) physical medicine specialists, and (13) ophthalmologists.

[8] Tennessee was not included as it did not have a Medicaid fee-for-service program. 9There was insufficient commercial data to analyze rates for obstetricians.

[10] The geographic market areas were equally distributed among the three TRICARE regions: two high-volume TRICARE markets and three smaller markets in each region.

[11] Kennell, D., Brooks, A., Witsberger, C., TRICARE Reimbursement of Pediatric Vaccines and Immunizations (Task Order No. 1005-005), Kennell and Associates, Inc. (Jan. 14, 2009).

[12] At the time of the study, TRICARE reimbursed providers for pediatric vaccines in two components: (1) a reimbursement for the vaccine and (2) a separate amount (in many cases) for the administration of the vaccine.

[13] Network providers may agree to accept lower reimbursements as a condition of network participation.

[14] According to the study, TRICARE payments for pediatric vaccines could not be compared to Medicaid payments because pediatric vaccines were typically supplied free to pediatricians by states and/or the Centers for Disease Control and Prevention's Vaccines for Children program. The Vaccines for Children program provides free vaccines to enrolled public and private providers for recommended immunizations for children who are Medicaid-eligible, uninsured, on Medicaid, American Indian/Alaska Native, or underinsured by having insurance that does not cover routine immunizations. When a pediatrician receives Vaccines for Children products free, he or she is usually paid an administration fee by most Medicaid programs which generally ranges between $3 and $10, with most states paying between $4 and $6. TRICARE's 2008 reimbursement rate for this same service is $20.57.

[15] Kennell and Associates, Inc., Analysis of TRICARE Payment Rates for Maternity/Delivery Services, Evaluation and Management Services, and Pediatric Immunizations (Mar. 30, 2006).

[16] The study examined the 14 maternity/delivery CPT codes with the highest number of TRICARE purchased care uses, as well as the most frequently billed CPT code under TRICARE used by pediatricians—a mid-level office visit for an established patient.

[17] The study examined the 2006 state Medicaid rates for 45 states. According to the study, Tennessee and Delaware did not have fee-for-service Medicaid programs at the time of the study, and Massachusetts, Rhode Island, and Kansas' data were unavailable.

[18] The study examined the median commercial rates for September 2005 in the 50 areas with the highest number of TRICARE purchased care deliveries in fiscal year 2005.

[19] Three of the four states in which the Medicaid rates exceeded TRICARE's reimbursement rates for this service were states that also had higher Medicaid rates for maternity/delivery services. The fourth state had Medicaid rates that were roughly equal to TRICARE's reimbursement rate for this service.

[20] See 10 U.S.C. §§ 1079(h)(1), 1086(f).

End Notes for Appendix III

[1] 32 C.F.R. § 199.14(j)(1)(iv)(D) (2010). According to a TMA official, TMA usually defines a locality using one or more zip codes.

[2] 32 C.F.R. § 199.14(j)(1)(iv)(E) (2010). 332 C.F.R. § 199.14(j)(1)(iv)(C) (2010).

End Notes for Appendix IV

[1] The federal responsibility for health care in Alaska includes, but is not limited to, providing or funding health care to users of the Indian Health Service, Medicare, Medicaid, TRICARE, and Veterans Health Administration.

[2] See Sebelius, Kathleen, Secretary of Health and Human Services, Report to Congress of the Interagency Access to Health Care in Alaska Task Force (Sept. 17, 2010, p. 19).

[3] Alaska ranks first in the nation in the percent of population receiving TRICARE or Veterans Health Administration paid services. The national average is about 4 percent of the population. See Report to Congress of the Interagency Access to Health Care in Alaska Task Force (Sept. 17, 2010, p.19).

[4] Alaska Center for Rural Health, Alaska's AHEC Institute of Social and Economic Research, 2009 Alaska Health Workforce Vacancy Study (December 2009).

[5] TRICARE administration and management in each of the other 49 states was overseen by one of three regional contractors.

[6] See 75 Fed. Reg. 67,695 (Nov. 3, 2010).

[7] TMA calculated that, on average, the Department of Veterans Affairs reimbursement rates were 35 percent higher than TRICARE's rates in 2006, and 73 percent higher than Medicare's rates in Alaska. The 13 reimbursement waivers in Alaska are in addition to the demonstration project rate increases.

[8] The seven measures included: (1) the number of unique beneficiaries who received civilian care; (2) the number of unique civilian physicians who saw a TRICARE beneficiary; (3) the number of services (visits and other services) received by TRICARE patients; (4) the number of civilian emergency room visits; (5) the number of visits and admissions by Alaska residents outside of Alaska (prior to 2007, many beneficiaries had to be sent outside of Alaska for services because physicians would not treat them in Alaska); (6) the number of TRICARE waivers granted for active-duty servicemembers; and (7) survey information on whether physicians are willing to accept TRICARE Standard patients (this indicator of access is based on results of TMA surveys). These seven measures were developed in discussions with TMA and TRICARE Regional Office officials.

[9] See Patient Protection and Affordable Care Act, Pub. L. No. 111-148, § 10501(b), 124 Stat. 119, 993-94 (2010) (adding section 5104 to PPACA).

[10] See Report to Congress of the Interagency Access to Health Care in Alaska Task Force (Sept. 17, 2010).

End Notes for Appendix V

[1] TMA defines an "adequate network" as one that ensures that all access standards are continuously maintained in all TRICARE Prime Service Areas for the delivery of health care under TRICARE Prime and Extra.

[2] Among others, these time and distance standards set allowable travel and appointment wait times. Specifically, under normal circumstances, travel time may not exceed 30 minutes from home to primary care delivery site, or 1 hour from home for specialty care, unless a longer time is necessary because of the absence of providers (including providers not part of the network) in the area. Additionally, the wait time for an appointment for well-patient visits or specialty care referrals shall not exceed 4 weeks; for a routine visit, the wait time for an appointment shall not exceed 1 week; and for an urgent care visit the wait time for an appointment shall generally not exceed 24 hours. Office waiting times in nonemergency circumstances must not exceed 30 minutes, except when emergency care is being provided to patients and disrupts the normal schedule. See 32 C.F.R. § 199.17(p)(5) (2010).

In: Military Health Care
Editor: Brian M. Gagliardi

ISBN: 978-1-62417-339-4
© 2013 Nova Science Publishers, Inc.

Chapter 5

ABORTION SERVICES AND MILITARY MEDICAL FACILITIES*

David F. Burrelli

SUMMARY

In 1993, President Clinton modified the military policy on providing abortions at military medical facilities. Under the change directed by the President, military medical facilities were allowed to perform abortions if paid for entirely with non-Department of Defense (DOD) funds (i.e., privately funded). Although arguably consistent with statutory language barring the use of Defense Department funds, the President's policy overturned a former interpretation of existing law barring the availability of these services. On December 1, 1995, H.R. 2126, the FY1996 DOD appropriations act, became law (P.L. 104-61). Included in this law was language barring the use of funds to administer any policy that permits the performance of abortions at any DOD facility except where the life of the mother would be endangered if the fetus were carried to term or where the pregnancy resulted from an act of rape or incest. Language was also included in the FY1996 DOD Authorization Act (P.L. 104-106, February 10, 1996) prohibiting the use of DOD facilities in the performance of abortions. These served to reverse the President's 1993 policy change. Recent attempts to change or modify these laws have failed.

---

* This is an edited, reformatted and augmented version of Congressional Research Service, Publication No. 95-387, dated June 7, 2012.

Over the last three decades, the availability of abortion services at military medical facilities has been subjected to numerous changes and interpretations. Within the last 15 years, Congress has considered numerous amendments to effectuate such changes. Although Congress, in 1992, passed one such amendment to make abortions available at overseas installations, it was vetoed.

Abortions are generally not performed at military medical facilities in the continental United States. In addition, few have been performed at these facilities abroad for a number of reasons. First, the U.S. military follows the prevailing laws and rules of foreign countries regarding abortion. Second, the military has had a difficult time finding health care professionals in uniform willing to perform the procedure.

With the enactment of P.L. 104-61 and P.L. 104-106, these questions became moot, because now, neither DOD funds nor facilities may be used to administer any policy that provides for abortions at any DOD facility, except where the life of the mother may be endangered if the fetus were carried to term. Privately funded abortions at military facilities are permitted when the pregnancy was the result of an act of rape or incest.

In 2010, language was added to the Senate version of the FY2011 National Defense Authorization Act that would allow any DOD facilities to perform privately funded abortions. As noted, the military follows local laws and practices to the greatest extent possible. This potential change would not likely have much of an effect outside of the United States since nations that host large numbers of U.S. military personnel maintain legal restrictions on abortions. On September 21, 2010, and December 15, 2010, attempts were made to move this legislation to the Senate floor for a vote. However, due to disagreements over procedures, cloture votes were taken and failed. The House-passed version of this legislation does not contain language pertaining to abortion. The FY2011 National Defense Authorization Act became P.L. 111-383 without the Senate provision allowing military facilities to be used to perform abortions.

In 2011, attempts to expand coverage for cases of rape and incest and allow for privately funded abortion were blocked in the Senate.

Language in the Senate version of the National Defense Authorization Act for FY2013 would expand coverage of government-funded abortions for cases of rape and incest.

PURPOSE

The purpose of this report is to describe and discuss the provisions for providing abortion services to military personnel, their dependents, and other military health care beneficiaries at military medical facilities. The report describes the history of these provisions, with particular emphasis on legislative actions. Finally, this report discusses a number of proposals to modify the law as well as other related legislative and administrative actions.

ISSUE

Language in the Senate version of the National Defense Authorization Act for FY2013 would expand coverage of government-funded abortions for cases of rape and incest.[1] Current law only allows for government-funded abortions in cases where the life of the mother would be at risk is the fetus was carried to term. Current law allows for privately funded abortion at military medical facilities where the life of the mother would be at risk is the fetus was carried to term or in cases where the pregnancy is the result of rape or incest.

Shortly after his inauguration on January 20, 1993, President Clinton issued a memorandum on abortions at military hospitals. This memorandum directed a change in policy so that abortions could be performed at military medical facilities provided that the procedure was "privately funded." This memo stated that:

> Section 1093 of title 10 of the United States Code prohibits the use of Department of Defense ("DOD") funds to perform abortions except where the life of a women would be endangered if the fetus were carried to term. By memorandum of December 21, 1987, and June 21, 1988, DOD has gone beyond what I am informed are the requirements of the statute and has banned all abortions at U.S. military facilities, even where the procedure is privately funded. The ban is unwarranted. Accordingly, I hereby direct that you reverse the ban immediately and permit abortion services to be provided, if paid for entirely with non-DOD funds and in accordance with other relevant DOD policies and procedures.[2]

The issue at hand was how the language in Title 10 of the United States Code and the President's memo were to be interpreted. As the President's memorandum made obvious, this language has been subject to varying interpretations that allowed or denied abortion services. Specifically, Section 1093 stated:

> Funds available to the Department of Defense may not be used to perform abortions except where the life of the mother would be endangered if the fetus were carried to term.[3]

Although the President's interpretation of the language was arguably consistent with the letter of the law, critics contend that it countermanded the spirit of the statute and is overly broad. In other words, it is argued that the intent of this language was to prevent the DOD from providing abortion services. Proponents of the Clinton change argued that Congress allowed for exactly this type of interpretation. Proponents note that this interpretation was particularly important for eligible beneficiaries who are deployed overseas in areas where affordable and sanitary abortion services may not be available in the local economy.

Following the election of the 104th Congress, Democrats were replaced by Republicans as committee leaders. Representative Robert K. Dornan, the then-new Republican chairman of the Military Personnel and Compensation Subcommittee (the then-House National Security Committee), noted that one of his priorities "[was] barring abortions at overseas military hospitals, even if the patients pay for them."[4] On December 1, 1995, P.L. 104-61 was enacted. According to this law:

> Sec. 8119. None of the funds made available in this Act may be used to administer any policy that permits the performance of abortions at medical treatment or other facilities of the Department of Defense.
>
> Sec. 8119A. The provision of Section 8119 shall not apply where the life of the mother would be endangered if the fetus were carried to term, or the pregnancy is the result of an act of rape or incest.

On February 10, 1996, P.L. 104-106 was enacted. This law further limited that availability of abortion services:

> Sec. 738(b). RESTRICTION ON THE USE OF FACILITIES—No medical treatment facility or other facility of the Department of Defense may be used to perform an abortion except where the life of the mother would be endangered if the fetus were carried to term or in a case in which the pregnancy is the result of an act of rape or incest.[5]

Since then, efforts to modify the law pertaining to abortions have become a routine part of the legislative process. As noted above, language has been included in the Senate version of the FY2013 National Defense Authorization

Act that would expand the availability of government-funded abortion to cases where the pregnancy was the result of rape and incest.

In conclusion, under current law, 10 U.S.C. Section 1093, Performance of Abortions: Restrictions

> (a) Restriction on Use of Funds.—Funds available to the Department of Defense may not be used to perform abortions except where the life of the mother would be endangered if the fetus were carried to term.
>
> (b) Restriction on Use of Facilities.—No medical treatment facility or other facility of the Department of Defense may be used to perform an abortion except where the life of the mother would be endangered if the fetus were carried to term or in a case in which the pregnancy is the result of an act of rape or incest.

BACKGROUND

There appears to be no evidence of a formal service policy on abortions prior to 1970. Sources familiar with the issue at that time note that the availability of abortion services at military medical facilities varied by service, location, physician, and "command milieu." Each of the services approached the issue differently. The Air Force tended to be somewhat more liberal, while the Army and the Navy tended to be somewhat more conservative. Each facility also tended to follow the laws and regulations of the state within which it was located. Individual physicians ultimately had a say regarding whether or not they personally would provide such services. Finally, the commanders of various medical facilities may have had some effect on how and under what circumstances abortion services may have been provided. Commanders often lead by example without explicitly stating their own opinions or policies, or giving direct orders. Subordinates are acutely aware of their commander's approach to issues and often will integrate this approach into their own practice. In other words, a policy may exist without one ever being officially stated. Although formal policy may not exist, physicians also follow professional guidelines, as they interpret them, by practicing "good medicine." Thus, the decision to provide an abortion may have been based on a host of medical indications particular to any given case. Generally, it appears that military physicians performed relatively few abortions at military medical facilities in this era.

In certain situations, such as in Vietnam (1961-1975), military medical facilities generally did not provide abortion services. Instead, medical evacuations to other countries that had available procedures (Japan, for example) provided access to abortion services.

In 1970, the office responsible for health affairs at DOD reportedly issued "orders that military hospitals perform abortions when it is medically necessary or when the mental health of the mother is threatened."[6] The rules, however, did not require military personnel to perform abortions. These rules were less restrictive than the abortion laws in a number of states. One year later, then-President Richard M. Nixon directed that military policy concerning abortions at military bases in the United States "be made to correspond with the laws of the States where the bases are located."[7] This correspondence of policy between the military and states (including foreign nations) came to be known as "the good neighbor policy."

Following the 1973 Supreme Court case of *Roe v. Wade*,[8] the Department of Defense funded abortions for any women eligible for DOD health care, subject to certain limitations: first, two physicians were required to find that the abortion was "medically indicated" or required for "reasons of mental health"; second, the funding for these services could not be in conflict with the law of the state in which the abortion is carried out.[9] Since states had differing rules regarding abortion, it was possible for women to be treated differently depending on the location of the facility. Nevertheless, there remains anecdotal evidence of variations in accessibility similar to those that existed before *Roe v. Wade*.

In 1975, concerns were raised over inconsistencies between state statutes and the *Roe* decision. Military medical personnel were instructed to follow the constitutional guidance provided in *Roe* in certain instances, even though the state statutes had not been successfully challenged in court.[10]

From August 31, 1976, to August 31, 1977, approximately 26,000 abortions were performed in military hospitals or in the CHAMPUS program.[11]

In 1978, an amendment to the Department of Defense appropriations bill offered by Representative Robert Dornan prohibited the use of Defense Department funds for abortions with certain exceptions. This amendment, as enacted, stated that:

> None of the funds appropriated by this Act shall be used to perform abortions except where the life of the mother would be endangered if the fetus were carried to term; or except for such medical procedures necessary

for the victims of rape or incest, when such rape or incest has been reported promptly to a law enforcement agency or public health service; or except in those instances where severe and long-lasting physical health damage to the mother would result if the pregnancy were carried to term when so determined by two physicians. Nor are payments prohibited for drugs or devices to prevent implantation of the fertilized ovum, or for medical procedures necessary for the termination of an ectopic pregnancy.[12]

In 1979, similar language was enacted in the FY1980 DOD appropriations act. The 1979 language did not contain any restrictions with regard to the "severe and long-lasting physical health damage to the mother that would result if the pregnancy were carried to term when so determined by two physicians." In other words, a determination that carrying the pregnancy to term would affect the physical health of a woman was not a basis for providing abortions under this language.[13]

This language did not prevent all abortions at military hospitals. Military hospitals overseas reportedly performed approximately 1,300 abortions in FY1979. These abortions were privately paid for. Defense officials allowed these procedures under the rationale that at certain overseas (or isolated U.S.) stations, safe and reliable civilian facilities were not always available.[14]

In 1980, the language included in the FY1981 DOD appropriations act was again modified as follows:

> None of the funds appropriated by this Act shall be used to perform abortions except where the life of the mother would be endangered if the fetus were carried to term; or except for such medical procedures necessary for the victim of rape or incest, when such rape has within seventy-two hours been reported to a law enforcement agency or public health service; nor are payments prohibited for drugs or devices to prevent implantation of the fertilized ovum, or for medical procedures necessary for the termination of an ectopic pregnancy: *Provided, however,* That the several States are and shall remain free not to fund abortions to the extent that they in their sole discretion deem appropriate.[15]

Under this language, the reporting requirement for incest was removed. Also, victims of rape were required to report the incident within 72 hours.[16] In addition, language was added encouraging the states to exercise their authority with regard to funding abortions.

The language was shortened considerably in 1981. Many of the exceptions to the prohibition of funding were removed. This language stated that:

> None of the funds provided by this Act shall be used to perform
> abortions except where the life of the mother would be endangered if the
> fetus were carried to term.[17]

Identical language was included in the following two years'
appropriations acts.[18] Finally, in 1984, Congress codified this language in Title
10, United States Code (see quoted text at the top of page 1).[19]

In 1988, DOD modified its rules to require a physician's statement for
abortion claims made via CHAMPUS. This change was instituted to assure
that all claims for abortions performed in the private sector and covered by
CHAMPUS were for life-threatening situations. "CHAMPUS officials said
life-threatening conditions include leukemia, breast cancer and other
malignancies, kidney failure, congestive heart failure, severe heart disease,
uncontrolled diabetes and several other conditions."[20]

On June 21, 1988, Dr. William Mayer, then-Assistant Secretary of
Defense (Health Affairs), issued a memorandum barring abortions in military
medical. Although Dr. Mayer recognized that privately paid abortions did not
violate the letter of the law, he issued the memorandum to avoid the
appearance of "insensitivity to the spirit" of the law.[21]

In 1990, an attempt to overturn this restriction failed. An amendment (to
the DOD authorization act) to allow abortions at military medical facilities
overseas was withdrawn when the Senate fell two votes short of the number
needed to invoke cloture (58-41).[22] The House of Representatives rejected a
similar amendment.

On May 22, 1991, the House of Representatives reversed itself and passed
(220-208) an amendment to the DOD authorization act that would have
reinstated the pre-paid overseas policy. Proponents argued that the language
would be merely a return to the policy as it existed prior to Dr. Mayer's memo
of 1988. Opponents countered that, as drafted, the amendment offered by
Representative AuCoin would go beyond the then-prevailing policy by
allowing abortions for any reason and at any time during the pregnancy.[23] The
measure was rejected once again when the Senate fell two votes short of the 60
votes needed to invoke cloture (58-40).[24]

The battle over this language intensified. Proponents stated that military
women or dependents overseas were forced into dangerous or life-threatening
situations in countries where safe, legal, or affordable abortions could not be
provided. Opponents argued that no woman was denied military transportation
to receive access to an abortion in another country.

Again in 1992, Representative AuCoin introduced language to overturn the restrictions on abortions at overseas military facilities. This amendment was passed (216-193).[25] On September 18, 1992, the Senate rejected (36-55) an effort to strike language overturning the restrictions on overseas abortions. Despite these votes, it was expected that President George H. W. Bush would veto any defense legislation reinstating the former policy. This expected veto was cited as the reason for the language being dropped by the conferees.[26] By unanimous consent, the Senate agreed to substitute the language pertaining to overseas abortions into S. 3144 after striking all after the enacting clause.[27] S. 3144 was simultaneously passed by unanimous consent. The House subsequently passed the measure (220-186) on October 3, 1992.[28]

Arguably, the Senate and House agreed to remove this language from the DOD authorization act in anticipation of a presidential veto. By removing the language and passing it as a free-standing bill, the authorization act was not jeopardized. Since this was not presented in the authorization act, it remains unknown whether President Bush would have exercised his veto authority over the entire bill. Nevertheless, President Bush did pocket-veto S. 3144 on October 31, 1992 (after the congressional adjournment). No attempt was made to override this veto.[29]

As a result of President Clinton's 1993 memorandum (see page 1), then-Secretary of Defense Les Aspin directed the secretaries of the military departments to reinstate the pre-1988 policy concerning the availability of abortions overseas. On May 9, 1994, the Assistant Secretary of Defense (Health Affairs), Dr. Stephen C. Joseph, released a memorandum[30] seeking to unify and make consistent DOD policy. This policy had five parts that (1) provided access to abortion services for service women and eligible dependents overseas, (2) required the valid consent of a parent or other designated person in the case of a minor who was "not mature enough and well enough informed to give valid consent," (3) relieved those medical practitioners directly involved from performing abortions if they objected, (4) respected host nation laws regarding abortion, and, (5) directed the Military Health Services System to provide other means of access if providing pre-paid abortion services at a facility was not feasible. Such alternate means could include supplementing staff with contract personnel, referrals, travel, etc. The cost of an abortion had been reported to be about $500.[31] (It should be noted that cost determination is not based on the actual cost of the service to the military but rather on estimates. As a result of the way DOD funds accounts, i.e., personnel, construction, operations and maintenance, etc., it is difficult to determine the valid cost of any one procedure. This has led some to question whether or not any federal funds are used in cases of "pre-paid" abortions.)

In practice, the policy instituted by President Clinton's 1993 action may not have had the effects the President had expected. Although abortion access had been liberalized in terms of overall policy, liberalization had not necessarily occurred in terms of actual access.

> In the six years preceding the 1988 ban, military hospitals overseas had performed an average of 30 abortions annually. Last spring, though, when the military medical officials surveyed 44 Army, Navy and Air Force obstetricians and gynecologists stationed in Europe, they found that all but one doctor adamantly refused to perform the procedure.
>
> That one holdout, too, quickly switched positions.... No military medical personnel willing to perform abortions have stepped forward in the Pentagon's sprawling Pacific theater of operations, either.[32]

A number of reasons have been advanced to explain this general unwillingness by health care personnel in uniform to perform these procedures. First, fewer medical schools require or provide training in these techniques than was the case in the years immediately following the *Roe v. Wade* decision.[33] Second, it is widely thought that the military in general, and military physicians in particular, tends to be more conservative on social issues than many population cohorts. Even if training were made available it is unlikely that many would volunteer. Third, the social order on military posts tends to be very close-knit and hierarchical. A subordinate may choose not to "ruffle the feathers" of a superior over such a contentious issue. Thus, the social norms established by superiors in the military environment are likely to translate into action or inaction by subordinates. This conventional wisdom gains credibility given the enormous amount of leverage superiors in the military have over the careers of subordinates. (Although this is true in the civilian context, it apparently exists to a lesser degree, especially in professional fields such as medicine in which civilians are generally unwilling to formally judge or second-guess professional colleagues.) Fourth, the medical team must consist of volunteers. Any member of a medical team needed to perform an abortion can essentially "veto" it. Fifth, since military physicians are paid a salary, and not on the basis of procedures performed, there is no economic incentive to provide abortions. Finally, rules exist requiring the services to respect the prevailing laws in each country. Thus, the restrictions of a particular country may limit the access to pre-paid abortions at military facilities (see **Appendix**).[34]

Given these factors and considerations, it was reported that 27 abortions were performed at military hospitals worldwide in 1993[35] and 10 in 1994. All of the 1994 abortions were reported to be "life of the mother" cases; that is, none were "pre-paid." According to data provided by the military services, the following table displays the number of therapeutic abortions by year by service:

Table 1. Therapeutic Abortions at Military Treatment Facilities

	1996	FY 97	FY 98	FY 99	FY 00	FY 01	FY 02	FY 03	FY 04	FY 05	FY 06	FY 07	FY 08	FY 09	TOTAL
Army[a]	4	3	1	1	0	4	4	3	3	4	1	2	3	1	34
Navy[b]									4	2	2	2	3	1	14
Air Force[c,d]	1	1	0	1	0	1	0	0	0	0	1	0	0	0	5
TOTAL	5	4	1	2	0	5	4	3	7	6	4	4	6	2	53

Source: Department of Defense.

Notes:

[a] ICD-9 Code Ranges: 635-636. Data Source Standard Inpatient Data Record (SIDR). All cases have been reviewed and determined to be within compliance of Federal law.

[b] ICD-9 Code Ranges: 635-636. No encounters for 636. Data source is the Standard Inpatient Data Record (SIDR) in the MHS Mart (M2) database. Data in M2 is truncated at FY04 and historic data prior to FY04 is unavailable. MHS Coding Guidelines changed 1 July 2006; those cases identified before 2006 will be pulled and analyzed to insure that they were coded using the policies in place prior to the coding guideline change.

[c] 1996 is different because the only information available was one cover sheet/narrative summary/operation report on an Active Reserve member.

[d] Data from 1997 forward was retrieved from the Biometric Data Quality Assurance.

(Since 2010, DOD has not responded to CRS requests for data on abortions.)

Over these 15 years, DOD has performed an average of 3.79 therapeutic abortions per year.

Responding to the lack of medical personnel willing to perform abortions, the Army's 7th Medical Command (Europe) sought in 1993 to hire a civilian physician whose duties would include providing abortion services.[36] This move would have been consistent with the President's memo stating that "[i]n circumstances in which it is not feasible to provide pre-paid abortion services in a particular military facility, the [Military Health Services System] shall develop other means to assure access." Such an affirmative step would have provided access where none was available before. However, such a step could have been viewed as encouraging abortion and threatened to provoke protests both within the uniformed services and in the international community.[37] To date, reports of protests have not been found.

Another consideration along similar lines is to expand the use of foreign physicians, as suggested by the Defense Advisory Committee for Women in the Services (DACOWITS). This may be effective in certain situations, but not all, since DOD is still required, as a result of the "good neighbor policy," to observe local laws. Countries such as Spain, South Korea, and Panama outlaw or sharply restrict abortions.[38]

Following German unification, in 1993, a German court issued an injunction against a law that would have unified abortion policies in the east and west. The *Bundestag*, lower house of the German parliament, struggled to write new laws. During this void, the performance of abortions or restrictions on abortion services at military facilities in Germany, although not illegal, may have been inflammatory to certain German sensitivities.[39] On August 21, 1995, German President Roman Herzog signed into law a measure passed by the *Bundestag* (on June 29) and approved by the *Bundesrat*, upper house (on July 14). Under this law, abortions are illegal (except in cases of rape or "medical necessity"), but a woman who seeks an abortion during the first 12 weeks of pregnancy will not be subject to criminal prosecution provided she attends a compulsory counseling session reviewing her options.[40]

Contracting with foreign physicians poses its own problems. Countries that lack professional medical personnel trained to U.S. standards (the very reason argued for providing these services in the first place) are less likely to have physicians with a skill level that would be commendable for contracting.

In certain cases, contracting may be an option, but it raises other considerations. If the patient was to pay the cost of the abortion, does such a cost include a pro-rated amount based on contracting, training, travel, and other costs required to provide these services? Inclusion of these in such a cost calculation could well make the price of these services prohibitive. Conversely, using Defense Department funds to make available "pre-paid" abortions (i.e., through contracting, travel, etc.) could be viewed as in conflict with 10 U.S.C. 1093.

According to a DOD Information Paper, in August 1994, "a policy on hiring non-military physicians to perform abortions was issued with specific reference to treatment facilities in Germany. DOD respects host nation laws regarding abortion."[41]

Furthermore, it was unlikely that abortion services would become more available if the military reduced the number of physicians as part of downsizing of the force structure. One drawdown proposal suggests that DOD could reduce the number of physicians in uniform by as much as 50%.[42] Under the Administration's long-term defense spending plans, 5,600 civilian medical personnel will be cut from the Army over the next six years. The Navy and Air Force, together, are expected to be reduced by less than 2,000. These reductions "amount to the equivalent of shutting three of the Army's eight medical centers, experts say."[43] The reduction of civilian professionals in the U.S. military may require DOD to rotate uniformed physicians back to the United States from overseas, further reducing the number of physicians overseas. Such a reduction would likely serve to reduce the availability of abortion services overseas.

On May 29, 2002, a federal judge ruled that the military must pay for a 1994 abortion of an anencephalic fetus.[44] Later, in August 2002, a second federal court ruled likewise in a separate case involving another anencephalic fetus.[45] Both cases were reversed on appeal.[46]

"PLAN B" AND RU-486

In February 2002, the DOD Pharmacy and Therapeutics (P&T) Executive Council recommended adding levonorgestrel, aka "Plan B," to the Basic Core Formulary,[47] subject to further review. Plan B is described as an emergency contraceptive used to prevent pregnancy following a known or suspected contraceptive failure (e.g., broken condom) or when a pregnancy may result because no contraception was used (e.g., rape). It is noted that it will not terminate an "established pregnancy." In other words, it is not RU-486, a known abortifacient, which chemically induces an abortion. RU-486 is subject to restrictions under 10 U.S.C. Section 1093.[48]

According to a DOD Information Paper, Plan B could possibly "prevent a pregnancy by interfering with ovulation, sperm transport through cervical mucus and fallopian tubes, release of pituitary gonadotropins, corpus luteum functions, fertilization, *embryo transport and implantation.*"[49] [emphasis added] The possibility of preventing a fertilized egg from implanting leads to the argument, for those who maintain that life begins at conception, that Plan

B represents a potential form of abortion in certain cases. In May 2002, the P&T Executive Council Meeting released the following:

> At the February 2002 DOD Pharmacy & Therapeutics (P&T) Executive Council meeting, the Council recommended the addition of levonorgestrel 0.75 mg (Plan B) to the Basic Core Formulary (BCF), subject to the review of the Director, TRICARE Management Activity (TMA) and/or the Assistance Secretary of Defense for Health Affairs (ASD(HA)). On 28 March 2002, the Executive Director of TMA signed an Action Memo approving the recommendation. On April 3, 2002 the co-chair of the DOD P&T Committee informed the Council members and pharmacy consultants of the decision, and re-informed the Council on 7 May 2002. On 8 May 2002 the Executive Council was reconvened briefly to announce that the Council co-chairs had been informed that the ASD(HA) also wanted to review the Council's recommendation and that the Executive Director of TMA had rescinded his earlier approval. Therefore, Plan B has NOT been approved for addition to the BCF at this time, and the ASD(HA) is reviewing the Council's recommendation. [Military Treatment Facilities] MTFs are required to include all BCF drugs on their local formularies. As a result of Plan B's removal from the BCF, each MTF's P&T committee must now re-evaluate whether this product is within the scope of practice at the MTF and whether the MTF wants to continue to have Plan B on its formulary.[50]

In May 2005, a proposed amendment to make Plan B available on all military bases died in the House Rules Committee (as part of its consideration of the FY2005 National Defense Authorization Act).[51] This is not to say that Plan B was not available at certain military bases or to military health care beneficiaries. On September 7, 2005, it was reported that certain military bases do have Plan B on hand and have offered it, usually in cases of sexual assault, but also in cases where other contraceptives failed or unprotected sex was involved. Further, military physicians may prescribe the medication allowing the beneficiary to have the prescription filled at civilian pharmacies.[52]

Although tangentially relevant to DOD policy, Plan B was the subject of controversy within the Food and Drug Administration (FDA):

> FDA Commissioner Lester Crawford on August 26 [2005] said the agency is indefinitely deferring Barr Laboratories' application for nonprescription sales of its emergency contraceptive Plan B and opening a 60-day public comment period on the application sparking charges that the decision was motivated by politics rather than science, ... FDA in May 2004 issued a "not approvable" letter in response to Barr's original application to

allow Plan B – which can prevent pregnancy if taken within 72 hours of sexual intercourse – to be sold without a doctor's prescription and in January delayed a ruling on Barr's revised application, which would allow EC to be sold without a doctor's prescription only to women ages 17 and older. During a confirmation hearing in March, Crawford told the Senate committee that FDA would approve the application "within weeks."[53]

On August 24, 2006, the FDA approved over-the-counter sales of Plan B to women 18 years old and older.[54] Nearly three months later, Plan B began appearing in drug stores.[55]

Although this latter controversy was not directly related to the Department of Defense, it appears that the decision made by the FDA was taken into consideration by DOD officials with regard to emergency contraceptives.

In 2007, according to the DOD Pharmacoeconomic Center, Plan B was not on the Basic Core Formulary, but Military Treatment Facilities may have had it on hand as part of their formulary.[56]

In June 2009, Plan B was voluntarily discontinued by the manufacturer and replaced by a product under the name "Next Choice."

In November 2009, P&T Committee recommended placing Next Choice on the BCF. On February 3, 2010, this recommendation was approved by TMA and Next Choice was placed on the list of drugs all military facilities stock.[57]

"PARENTAL NOTIFICATION"

"Parental notification" is concerned with those instances in which an abortion is sought at a military facility by or on behalf of a military dependent who is a minor and/or incapable of making such a decision.

According to DOD:

> Assuming that an abortion is authorized [under statute], consent must be obtained before any surgical procedure is performed. The requirement to obtain consent is required in military treatment facilities (MTFs), because the standard of care for medical practice in MTFs within the United States is governed by the Federal Tort Claims Act (FTCA). The standard of care for obtaining consent under FTCA is that the provider will follow state law governing the circumstances under which a minor may consent for medical treatment. In overseas facilities, consent by minors for abortions is governed by [DOD] Health Affairs Policy dated May 9, 1994, as amended by [DOD]

Health Affairs Policy 96-030, dated February 13, 1996. Those policies state that the host nation laws or legal requirements will apply. In the absence of such host nation laws or legal requirements, valid consent for minors may be obtained in either of two methods. First, the consent of at least one parent or guardian is provided. Second, the commanding officer of the medical treatment facility (or if the commanding officer is not a physician, a senior physician designated by the commanding officer) makes a judgment, upon the recommendation of the attending physician, that the minor is mature enough and well enough informed to give valid consent, or, if she is not sufficiently mature and informed, that the desired abortion would be in her best interest.[58]

LEGISLATIVE ACTION SINCE 1995

The House version of the FY1996 Defense Authorization Act contained a section that would terminate the policy of allowing the performance of abortions on a pre-paid basis, at military facilities. Under this language:

> This section would amend Section 1093 of Title 10, United States Code, to include restricting the Department of Defense from using medical treatment facilities or other DOD facilities, as well as DOD funds, to perform abortions unless necessary to save the life of the mother.[59]

The Senate report contained no similar provisions.

As a result of numerous political differences between the House and the Senate language, as well as Administration opposition on a number of issues raising the specter of a veto, the authorization act stalled in conference. Legislators sought to have language included in the FY1996 DOD appropriations act that would prohibit abortions at overseas military facilities. The Appropriations Conference Committee originally included the following language:

> Sec. 8119. None of the funds made available in this Act may be used to administer any policy that permits the performance of abortions at medical treatment or other facilities of the Department of Defense, except when it is made known to the federal official having authority to obligate or expend such funds that the life of the mother would be endangered if the fetus were carried to term: Provided, That the provisions of this section shall enter into force if specifically authorized in the National Defense Authorization Act for Fiscal Year 1996.

Thus, the nature of this language only allowed it to take effect, when and if the authorization language was enacted into law. As noted, at the time, the authorization bill was stalled in conference and faced a possible veto. The failure of the authorization bill to be passed would negate any language concerning abortions in the appropriations bill.

On September 29, 1995, pro-life legislators in the House and a large number of Democrats (opposed to the bill on policy and other spending considerations) joined ranks and rejected the conference version of the FY1996 DOD appropriations act (151-267), thereby returning the bill to the House-Senate conference.[60] On November 16, 1995, the conferees agreed to a compromise that included the following language:

> Sec. 8119. None of the funds made available in this Act may be used to administer any policy that permits the performance of abortions at medical treatment or other facilities of the Department of Defense.
> Sec. 8119A. The provision of Section 8119 shall not apply where the life of the mother would be endangered if the fetus were carried to term, or the pregnancy is the result of an act of rape or incest.

On December 1, 1995, the appropriations act, with the above two sections, became law.[61]

On December 15, 1995, the House passed the FY1996 Authorization Act (containing the language cited on page 13). The bill was approved by the Senate on December 19, 1995. On December 28, 1995, the President vetoed the authorization act, and in a letter to Congress, he stated:

> H.R. 1530 [FY1996 Defense Authorization Act] also contains ... provisions that would unfairly affect certain service members.... I remain very concerned about provisions that would restrict service women and female dependents of military personnel from obtaining privately funded abortions in military facilities overseas, except in the cases of rape, incest, or danger to the life of the mother. In many countries, these U.S. facilities provide the only accessible, safe source for these medical services. Accordingly, I urge Congress to repeal a similar provision that became law in the "Department of Defense appropriations act, 1996.[62]

On January 3, 1996, the House of Representatives failed to override the veto with a vote of 240- 156. Two days later, the House amended S. 1124 by striking "all after the enacting clause of S. 1124 and insert[ing] in lieu thereof the text of H.R. 1530 [the vetoed language] as reported by the committee of conference on December 13, 1995, contained in [H. Rept. 104-406]."[63] Under unanimous consent, the language was taken from the Speaker's table, as amended, and sent to conference. On January 22, conference report H.Rept. 104-450 was filed. On January 24, 1996, the House agreed to the conference report (287-129). Two day later, the Senate agreed to the conference report (56-34). Provisions barring the use of DOD facilities to perform abortions, except in cases of rape, incest or where the life of the mother would be endangered if the fetus were carried to term or in a case in which the pregnancy, were included in this language (see quoted text on page 2). On February 10, 1996, President Clinton signed the FY1996 Defense Authorization Act into law.[64]

Although the prohibition against using funding in the appropriations act would have lapsed at the end of the fiscal year, the change made via the authorization act modifies Title 10 United States Code. As such, this change will not lapse at the end of the fiscal year. Thus, this language will stay in effect unless and until Congress (with the President's signature) specifically acts to amend, modify, strengthen or repeal these provisions.

On May 14, 1996, an amendment was offered to the House version of the FY1997 National Defense Authorization Act to overturn the prohibition on military facilities performing abortions and allow such abortions to be performed at these medical facilities so long as federal funds are not used (i.e., patient-paid abortions). The amendment was defeat by a vote of 192 ayes and 225 noes.[65] Slightly more than one month later, the Senate passed an identical amendment to its version of the FY1997 National Defense Authorization Act by a voice vote.[66] Ultimately, the Senate conferees receded and the Senate amendment was dropped.

Efforts to amend these provisions have continued. On June 19, 1997, Representative Jane Harman offered an amendment to the FY1998 DOD Authorization Act that would purportedly

> [restore the] policy affording access to certain health care procedures for female members of the armed forces and dependents at Department of Defense facilities.

The amendment was rejected (196-224).[67]

In 1998, the House National Security Committee rejected another attempt to allow for privately funded abortions at these facilities.[68] On June 25, 1998, the Senate rejected a similar provision (44-49).[69]

During consideration of the FY2000 National Defense Authorization Act, the House Personnel Subcommittee accepted an amendment by Representative Loretta Sanchez to reverse the restrictions on privately funded abortions being performed at overseas military medical facilities. Another amendment, by Representative Kuykendall, would have allowed Defense Department funding of abortions in cases of rape or incest. Upon consideration by the House Armed Services Committee, the Sanchez amendment was dropped and the Kuykendall amendment was further amended by Representative Buyer. As amended, the Kuykendall amendment would allow Defense Department funding of abortions in cases of *forcible* rape or incest *provided that the rape or incest had been reported to a law enforcement agency.* [Italics represent the Buyer changes.] Later efforts to reinstate the Sanchez language allowing for abortions at overseas military facilities when personal funds are used were rejected by both the House and the Senate. Ultimately, the Kuykendall amendment, as amended, was also deleted during conference consideration of the FY2000 National Defense Authorization Act, thereby leaving the law unchanged.[70]

Although not specifically related to the above discussion of the military abortion issue, other language has been proposed that would have had an effect on the consideration of the abortion issue. H.R. 2436[71] included, in part, language modifying Title 10, United States Code. According to this language, any conduct violating certain provisions of the Uniform Code of Military Justice, by a person subject to the Uniform Code of Military Justice, that causes death or bodily injury to a fetus who is in utero at the time the conduct takes place, would be guilty of a criminal offense. For example, if during an assault on a pregnant women, the fetus were injured, such an injury would constitute a separate offense. Exceptions were included in cases of abortions, medical treatment of the woman, or conduct of the woman with regard to her fetus. On September 30, 1999, the House passed this language (254-172). The next day, it was received and read in the Senate. On February 23, 2000, the Senate Committee on Judiciary held hearings on a Senate companion bill, S. 1673. No further action was then taken by the Senate, and the legislation failed to become law. (Similar language was considered in 2004; see "Unborn Victims of Violence Act 2004," below.)

Proponents note that such language would recognize the victimization of the child while in utero and afford appropriate criminal sanctions to perpetrators of violent acts. Critics view the inclusion of such language as a means of defining a fetus as a victim and thereby acknowledging or creating a separate human existence. These critics are concerned that such language would arguably recognize the fetus as separate person in the eyes of the law thereby complicating the abortion debate.[72]

In consideration of the FY2001 National Defense Authorization Act (H.R. 4205), the House Armed Services Committee "voted to retain its ban on abortions at military hospitals unless the mother's life is at risk. The 31-20 vote came May 10, 2000, on an amendment that would have allowed abortions at overseas hospitals if patients rather than the government paid for them. The 29-26 vote came on a failed try to allow military hospitals to perform abortions in cases of rape or incest."[73] Eight days later, a floor amendment was offered that would strike subsections a and b of 10 U.S.C. Section 1093, effectively removing any restriction to providing abortions under this title. The amendment was defeated (221-195).[74]

On June 20, 2000, the Senate tabled (50-49) an amendment to the FY2001 National Defense Authorization Act, S. 2549, that would strike Section b of 10 U.S.C. Section 1093. The amendment would have lifted the ban on the use of military facilities in performing abortions. Although proponents noted that the amendment "would lift restrictions on privately funded abortions at military facilities overseas," as written, the amendment would affect such facilities in the United States as well.[75]

On September 25, 2001, Representative Loretta Sanchez offered an amendment to the National Defense Authorization Act for FY2002. This amendment would have limited the restriction on the use of DOD facilities for performing abortions at those facilities "in the United States." In other words, this language would remove the restriction of providing privately funded abortion services at DOD facilities overseas. The amendment was rejected (199-217).[76]

During debate on the Bob Stump FY2003 National Defense Authorization Act, the Senate (52-40) passed an amendment that would remove the restriction on the use of military facilities.[77] The House had earlier rejected a similar measure (215-202).[78] In a letter to Senator Carl Levin, then-Chairman of the Armed Services Committee, Secretary of Defense Donald H. Rumsfeld wrote:

> The Senate bill removes the current statutory prohibition on access to abortion services at Department of Defense (DOD) medical facilities. The President's senior advisors would recommend that the President veto the bill if it changes current law.[79]

The Senate amendment was dropped by the conference committee.[80]

On April 1, 2004, President Bush signed H.R. 1997, "Unborn Victims of Violence Act of 2004 (Laci and Conner's Law)" into law.[81] Although intended to protect fetuses, this legislation contains a provision that would not permit the prosecution "of any person for conduct relating to an abortion" in which consent was legally obtained or implied.

Amendments to the FY2004 National Defense Authorization Act to modify the law were also offered. In the House, an amendment that would have limited the restriction on DOD facilities to the United States was rejected (201-227).[82]

Likewise the Senate rejected (48-51) an amendment that would have repealed the restriction on using DOD facilities, in general.[83]

However, the Senate agreed, subject to certain limitations, to consider legislation, S. 1104,[84] "to provide for parental involvement in abortions of dependent children of the Armed Forces." The legislation was placed on the Legislative Calendar[85] but failed to be called to the floor.

Consideration of the Ronald W. Reagan FY2005 National Defense Authorization Act included a number of amendments regarding abortion services. In the House of Representatives, Representative Susan A. Davis introduced an amendment that would allow military personnel and their dependents to use their own funds to obtain abortion services at overseas military hospitals. This amendment was defeated (202-221).[86]

In the Senate, an amendment offered by Senator Barbara Boxer, would allow DOD funding of abortions in cases of rape or incest. This amendment, along with 25 other amendments, was passed *en bloc* by unanimous consent.[87] On October 8, 2004, the conference report for this legislation noted that the "Boxer amendment" had been dropped.[88]

Two other Senate amendments to the Ronald W. Reagan FY2005 National Defense Authorization Act (H.R. 4200) were submitted. The first, S.Amdt. 3406 (Senators Frist and Brownback), would "provide for parental involvement in the performance of abortions for dependent children of members of the Armed Forces." The second, S.Amdt. 3407 (Senators Frist and Brownback), would require the notification of authorities regarding the identity of perpetrators, where possible, in cases of rape or incest when abortions are sought at military facilities. Neither S.Amdt. 3406 nor S.Amdt. 3407 was called up.

On May 25, 2005, the House of Representatives considered an amendment (offered by Representative Susan Davis) to the National Defense Authorization Act for Fiscal Year 2006 (H.R. 1815). The amendment would allow overseas military facilities to provide privately funded abortions for women who are in the miliary or are military dependents. This amendment was rejected (194-233).[89]

On July 25, 2005, Senator Lautenberg filed an amendment in the Senate that would "restore the previous policy regarding restrictions on the use of medical treatment facilities or other Department of Defense facilities." This amendment would strike Section 1093(b) of title 10 U.S.C. (and remove the title language "Restriction on Use of Funds.–" from Section 1093(a)). No further action has been taken on this amendment.[90]

On May 10, 2006, the House of Representatives considered an amendment (offered by Representative Robert E. Andrews) to the John Warner FY2007 National Defense Authorization Act that would allow overseas military facilities to provide privately funded abortions for women who are in the military or are military dependents. This amendment was rejected (191-237).

Recent Legislative Action

Language included in the Senate version of the National Defense Authorization Act for Fiscal Year 2011[91] would, if enacted, repeal the prohibition on using any military facilities to perform abortion, with certain exceptions. This action would allow the Department of Defense to return to the Clinton administration policy of allowing military facilities to provide abortions using private funds. Similar language was not included in the House version. On September 21, 2010, and December 15, 2010, attempts were made to move this legislation to the floor for a vote. However, due to disagreements over procedures, cloture votes were taken and failed. Ultimately, the FY2011 National Defense Authorization Act became P.L. 111-383 without the Senate provision allowing military facilities to be used to perform abortions.

Amendments to the National Defense Authorization Act for FY 2012, offered by Sen. Jeanne Shaheen, were not include in the final passed version. S.Amdt. 1120 would have expanded government-funded abortion at military medical facilities to include pregnancies resulting from rape or incest. S.Amdt. 1121 would have removed subsection 10 U.S.C. 1093(b) thereby allowing for a return to the Clinton policy of allowing privately funded abortions.[92]

As noted on page 1, it was reported that language had been included in the National Defense Authorization Act for FY 2013 that would allow for government-funded abortions in cases where the pregnancies resulted from rape or incest.

APPENDIX. AVAILABILITY OF ABORTION SERVICES AT MILITARY FACILITIES OVERSEAS

According to Department of Defense and individual command officials (as reported to the *Army Times*, September 5, 1994: 18; source: Defense Department and individual command officials), the availability of abortion services (prior to the restrictions enacted on December 1, 1995) at military facilities overseas could vary depending on location.

Germany

- **National policy:** See discussion on page 9 above.
- **Local U.S. military policy:** Under German law, abortions are illegal except in cases of rape or medical necessity. Abortions carried out during the first twelve weeks of pregnancy are not considered a prosecutable offense provided the woman has certification attesting to receiving state approved counseling to review her options. The military does not allow abortions at its facilities.
- **Since the U.S. ban was lifted:** Estimates of how many American service women or family members received abortions from German providers in 1993 are as high as 1,500, although German officials say there is no way to confirm this number.

Italy

- **National policy:** Abortions are permitted. They must be performed by a licensed gynecologist.
- **Local U.S. military policy:** Abortion services comparable to those in the United States are available from Italian providers in the Naples and Sigonella areas. Service women and family members who desire abortions are referred to pre-identified licensed local providers. Abortions are not performed at military hospitals.
- **Since the U.S. ban was lifted:** One elective abortion was reportedly provided in Sigonella at an Italian facility.

Japan

- **National policy:** Abortion is legal and fairly unrestricted, but more expensive than in the United States.
- **Local U.S. military policy:** Given that abortions are readily available in the Japanese community, women seeking abortion from Navy hospitals here are referred to family-service counselors for referrals to Japanese doctors.
- **Since the U.S. ban was lifted:** Few, if any, abortions were performed at military hospitals, Navy officials said. The number of abortions by civilian doctors is unknown.

Korea

- **National policy:** Abortion is illegal except to save the life of the mother. However, it has been noted that Korean women have not been denied access to medically provided abortion services despite this law.
- **Local U.S. military policy:** The U.S. military's rules for Korea could not be learned from military officials, but because of the local law, abortions would not be available at U.S. hospitals. However, since Korean women have access to such services, it is reasonable to infer that such services could also be available to U.S. service women off-base.
- **Since the U.S. ban was lifted:** Service members or family members continue to have to travel outside of Korea to obtain an abortion.

For a country-by-country listing of abortion laws and policies go to the following website: http://www.un.org/esa/population/publications/abortion/profiles.htm.

Problematic Comparisons to Foreign Military Policies

Abortion policies of foreign militaries vary. These variations depend on the country's general policy regarding abortion. For instance, abortion policies are affected by religion (Vatican, Israel, and Islamic nations, for example), population control policies (China) and other cultural factors (nationalized health care policies, such as are found in Great Britain), and issues pertaining to the structure of the military—the presence of women in uniform (many Islamic countries do not have women in uniform, making the issue moot). Some countries do not have a military (Costa Rica for instance does not have a military per se but rather a paramilitary style security force). In addition, internal legal restrictions or rulings, such as court rulings on abortion (see Germany), affect the country's policy. Finally, very few countries maintain a level of overseas deployments that make direct comparisons relevant. For these reasons, comparisons to foreign nations in terms of their abortion policy in general, and their policy regarding military abortions at overseas military medical facilities, in particular, are difficult to justify and of questionable utility.

End Notes

[1] Cunningham, Paige Winfield, "Abortion Funding Fight Could Complicate Defense Spending Legislation," *The Washington Times*, May 30, 2012: 7.

[2] President William J. Clinton, Memorandum for the Secretary of Defense, Memorandum on Abortions in Military Hospitals, January 22, 1993; filed with the Office of the Federal Register, 11:50 a.m., January 27, 1993; cited in Public Papers of the Presidents of the United States, William J. Clinton, 1993, Washington, D.C., Government Printing Office, 1994: 11.

[3] 10 U.S.C. Sec. 1093, added P.L. 98-525, Sec. 1401(e)(5), October 19, 1984, 98 Stat. 2617. It should be noted that the Civilian Health and Medical Program of the Uniformed Services (CHAMPUS, now TRICARE), a medical program for military dependents, certain retirees and their dependents who are unable to receive care at a military medical facility, will provide coverage for abortions only when the mother's life is in danger. "The attending physician must certify in writing that the abortion was performed because a life-endangering condition existed, and must provide medical documentation to the CHAMPUS claims processor in order for CHAMPUS to share the cost of the procedure." See U.S. Department of Defense, OCHAMPUS, CHAMPUS Handbook, October 1994: 42.

[4] Maze, Rick, "Representative Dornan: 'Pay gap one of top concerns,'" *Army Times*, January 16, 1995: 3.

[5] U.S. Congress, Conference Committee, National Defense Authorization Act for Fiscal Year 1996, H.Rept. 104-450, S. 1124, 104th Cong., 2nd Sess., January 22, 1996: 206-207.

[6] Wolffe, Jim, "Abortion ban may be lifted soon stateside," *Air Force Times*, April 12, 1993: 23.

[7] Statement about Policy on Abortions at Military Base Hospitals in the United States, April 3, 1971, Public Papers of the Presidents of the United States, Richard Nixon, 1971, Washington: GPO, 1972) p. 500. Since CHAMPUS (the point of service contract health care for non-active duty beneficiaries—now known as TRICARE Standard) relied, then as now, on local health care providers, these individuals were already subject to State laws and regulations pertaining to abortion.

[8] *Roe v. Wade*, 410 U.S. 113 (1973). The Court held that the Constitution protects a woman's decision whether or not to terminate pregnancy and that a State may not unduly burden the exercise of that fundamental right by regulations that prohibit or substantially limit access to the means of effectuating that decision.

[9] Ayres, B. Drummond, Jr., *New York Times*, August 10, 1978: 79 (microfilm).

[10] U.S. Department of Defense, Assistant Secretary of Defense (Health and Environment), James R. Cowen, Memorandum for the Assistant Secretaries of the Military Departments (M&RA), Abortion Policy, September 17, 1975.

[11] U.S. Department of Defense, Directorate for Defense Information, Press Division, 9 August, 1978.

[12] P.L. 95-457, §863, October 13, 1978, 92 Stat. 1254. In anticipation of this change, the Office of the Assistant Secretary of Defense (Public Affairs) published a News Release (September 29, 1978) functionally implementing this language effective September 30, 1978. This change also affected funding for CHAMPUS claims.

[13] P.L. 96-154, §762, December 21, 1979, 93 Stat. 1162.

[14] Smith, Paul, "1300 FY79 O'seas Abortions Revealed," *Army Times*, December 8, 1980: 2.

[15] P.L. 96-527, §760, December 15, 1980, 94 Stat. 3091.

[16] Previous language required that such a report should be made "promptly." DOD interpreted this to mean within 48 hours. It was also expected that victims of incest would report the incident(s) to appropriate authorities, however, the lack of a time restriction meant that a report could be delayed indefinitely. (See "DOD Issues New Rules On Abortion," *Army Times*, March 9, 1981: 15.)

[17] P.L. 97-114, §757, December 29, 1981, 95 Stat. 1588.

[18] P.L. 97-377, §755, December 21, 1982, 96 Stat. 1860; P.L. 98-212, §751, December 8, 1983, 97 Stat. 1447.

[19] 10 U.S.C. 1093, P.L. 98-525, sec 1401(e)(5), October 19, 1984, 98 Stat. 2617. Note this change occurred via an authorization act and not as a part of the appropriations process (*Omnibus Defense Authorization Act, 1985*).

[20] Kimble, Vesta, "Doctor's Statement Needed for Abortion Claims," *Navy Times*, March 14, 1988: 24.

[21] "Abortion Is Restricted At Military Hospitals," *New York Times*, July 19, 1988: A11. "The abortion issue in military hospitals has a symbolic and political importance that dwarfs the actual numbers of people involved. Military hospitals overseas performed only six abortions in the last year they were permitted [1987]." Willis, Grant, "Clinton Ends Ban on Military Abortions," *Air Force Times*, February 1, 1993: 4; and, U.S., Department of Defense, Assistant Secretary of Defense, William Mayer, M.D., Memorandum for Military Departments, DOD Policy Regarding Non-Funded Abortions in Outside the Continental United States Medical Treatment Facilities, June 21, 1988, "The policy is that the performance of pre-paid abortions in military treatment facilities is not authorized."

[22] Congressional Record, August 3, 1990: S11813-S11824.

[23] Congressional Record, May 22, 1991: H3394 et seq.

[24] Nelson, Soraya, "Overseas Abortion Amendment Fails," *Army Times* December 1991: 16.

[25] Congressional Record, June 4, 1992: H4150-H4156.

[26] Dewar, Helen, "Bush's Veto Power Stalled the Abortion-Rights Push in Congress," *Washington Post*, November 30, 1991: A6.

[27] Both House and Senate versions of the FY1993 Defense Authorization Act contained provisions that would "entitle military personnel and their dependents to reproductive health care services in a medical facility of the uniformed services outside the United States on a

reimbursement basis.... The conferees agree to exclude this provision. The Senate has passed a bill (S. 3144) that contains this provision. The House intends to pass this bill and send it to the President as soon as possible." U.S. Congress, House Conference Committee, National Defense Authorization Act for Fiscal Year 1993, H.Rept. 102-966, H.R. 5006, 102d Cong., 2nd Sess., October 1, 1992: 716.

[28] See H.Res. 589, Congressional Record, October 2, 1992: H10803-H10804, and Congressional Record, October 3, 1992: H10966-H10975.

[29] Congressional Quarterly, December 19, 1992: 3926.

[30] U.S. Department of Defense, Assistant Secretary of Defense (Health Affairs), Memorandum, Implementation of Policy Regarding Pre-Paid Abortions in Military Treatment Facilities, May 9, 1994: 2p.

[31] Nelson, Soraya S., "Pentagon Pens Rules on Abortion," Army Times, May 23, 1994: 10.

[32] Morrison, David C., "An Order That Didn't Take," National Journal, April 16, 1994: 900.

[33] According to the Alan Guttmacher Institute, from 1976 to 1991, the proportion of residency programs that did not offer abortion training rose from 7.5 to 31%. In 1976, 26% of the residency programs required abortion training. By 1991, only 12% required such training. The Accreditation Council for Graduate Medical Education has directed obstetrical residents should be taught how to perform abortions, unless they have a moral or religious objection. This change in policy was scheduled to become effective on January 1, 1996. Abortion mandated for OB training, Washington Times, February 15, 1995: A12. On March 19, 1996, the Senate passed the Coats amendment (no. 3513): "to amend the Public Health Service Act to prohibit governmental discrimination in the training and licensing of health professionals on the basis of the refusal to undergo or provide training in the performance of induced abortions," by a vote of 63 yeas and 37 nays. Congressional Record, March 19, 1996, S2262-S2266, S2268-S2276, S2280.

[34] "Most countries where American military personnel are stationed restrict or outlaw them [abortions] altogether." Nelson, Soraya S., "Limits Remain on Abortions at Overseas Hospitals," Navy Times, February 22, 1993: 11.

[35] Nelson, Soraya S., "Military Abortions Overseas: Still Rare," Army Times, September 5, 1994: 18.

[36] Scholar, Steve, "Army Seeking Civilian Doctor Willing To Do abortions at Military Hospitals," Stars and Stripes (European), April 28, 1993: 1.

[37] "A Pentagon Decision To Send Doctors Overseas To Perform Abortions in Military Hospitals Could Spark Protest from Pro-Life Groups in Germany, Pro-Life GIs say," Pro-Life Protests, American Legion, July 1994: 10.

[38] "Women in the services," Fast Track, Army Times, July 4, 1994: 20.

[39] "Women's groups, opposition politicians from the west, and easterners across the political spectrum expressed outrage at the court's decision. Many observers felt the decision exposed the deep east-west social divide." CRS Issue Brief IB91018, German-American Relations in the New Europe, by Karen E. Donfried, January 27, 1994, p. 6 (out-ofprint; available from the author at 7-8033).

[40] The Week in Germany, January 30, 1998.

[41] Memorandum for Assistant Secretary of Defense (Health Affairs), Information Paper on abortion policy for Dr. Hambre's confirmation hearing, July 1997.

[42] "In June [1994], a Pentagon study found that only about half of the current number of military doctors are needed for any foreseeable military operation." Jowers, Karen, "50% Cut Is Planned in Military Doctors," Air Force Times, January 23, 1995: 28.

[43] Nelson, Soraya S., "Medicare Users May Lose Hospital Access," *Navy Times*, September 5, 1994: 26.

[44] *Britell v. United States*, 204 F.Supp.2d 182, May 29, 2002.

[45] Ostrom, Carol M., "Judge: Navy Must Cover Women's Abortion," *Seattle Times*, August 13, 2002. The 9th Circuit Court of Appeals, without comment, denied a last minute appeal in this case. "Court Rejects Effort to Stop Navy Funding of Abortion," *Baltimore Sun*, August 18, 2002.

[46] *Britell v. United States*, 372 F.3d 1370, June 24, 2004, and *Doe v. USA*, et al., civil docket for case #: 2:02-cv-01657- TSZ, August 18, 2005.

[47] The Basic Core Formulary or BCF refers to those pharmaceuticals that DOD makes available at DOD pharmacies.

[48] Legislation was offered in the 109th Congress (S. 511, Senator DeMint, March 3, 2005 and H.R. 1079, Rep. Bartlett) "To provide that the approved application under the Federal Food, Drug, and Cosmetic Act for the drug commonly known as RU-486 is deemed to have been withdrawn, to provide for the review by the Comptroller General of the United States of the process by which the Food and Drug Administration approved such drug, and for other purposes." Both bills were referred to Committees and have received no further action.

[49] Col. Daniel Remund, Co-chair, DOD Pharmacy & Therapeutics Committee, Information Paper, April 11, 2002.

[50] Department of Defense, Pharmaeconomic Center, Minutes of the DOD Pharmacy & Therapeutics Executive Council Meeting, May 7, 2002, pp. 2-3.

[51] The proposal was similar to language contained in H.R. 2635, Rep. Michael H. Michaud, May 25, 2005.

[52] Montgomery, Nancy, Army Hospitals in Europe Offering 'Morning-After' Pill, *Stars and Stripes* (European edition), June 8, 2005.

[53] "FDA: Indefinitely Defers Decision on Emergency Contraceptive; Plan B," *National Journal Group, Inc.*, September 6, 2005

[54] Harris, Gardiner, F.D.A. Approves Broader Access t Next-Day Pill, *New York Times*, August 25, 2006: 1.

[55] Payne, January W., "For Plan B, A Broader Reach," *Washington Post*, November 21, 2006: F1.

[56] DOD, MTF Formulary Management For Contraceptives (Updated 26 Jan 07).

[57] Stein, Rob, "Pentagon to stock health facilities with morning-after pill," *The Washington Post*, February 5, 2010.

[58] Letter from Speight, Cynthia, CIV, OASD(HA)TMA to Richard Best, CRS, May 28, 2003.

[59] U.S. Congress, House Committee on National Security, National Defense Authorization Act for Fiscal Year 1996, H.Rept. 104-131, H.R. 1530, 104th Cong., 1st Sess., June 1, 1995: 237.

[60] Maze, Rick, and William Matthew, "Defense Spending Bill Slapped Back by Unlikely Union in Congress," *Army Times*, October 9, 1995: 25.

[61] P.L. 104-61, 109 Stat. 636, December 1, 1995.

[62] Veto message from the President of the United States (H. Doc. No. 104-155), cited in the Congressional Record, January 3, 1996: H12.

[63] Congressional Record, January 5, 1996: H302.

[64] P.L. 104-106, 110 Stat. 186, February 10, 1996.

[65] Congressional Record, May 14,1996, H5013-H5022.

[66] Congressional Record, June 19, 1996, S6460-S6469.

[67] Congressional Record, June 19, 1997, H4056-H4069.

[68] CQ Weekly, Other Policy Issues, May 9, 1998: 1240.

[69] Congressional Record, June 25, 1998, S7060-S7076.

[70] Maze, Rick, "Abortion Provision Dropped from Defense Bill," *Times*, August 16, 1999: 11.

[71] H.R. 2436, Representative Linsey Graham, July 1, 1999.

[72] For additional information on the legal aspects of the abortion issue, see CRS Report RL33467, *Abortion: Judicial History and Legislative Response*, by Jon O. Shimabukuro.

[73] FastTrack, *Times*, May 29, 2000: 6.

[74] Congressional Record, May 18, 2000: H3347-H3350, H3371.

[75] Congressional Record, June 20, 2000: S5406-S5421, S5425.

[76] Congressional Record, September 25, 2001: H6022-25, H6032-33.

[77] Congressional Record, June 21, 2002: S5882.

78 Congressional Record, May 9, 2002: H2380.

[79] Letter from Secretary of Defense Donald H. Rumsfeld to the Honorable Carl Levin, September 24, 2002.

[80] Congressional Record, November 12, 2002: H8462.

[81] P.L. 108-212; 1185 Stat. 568; April 1, 2004.

[82] Congressional Record, May 22, 2003: H4571.

[83] Congressional Record, May 22, 2003: S6911.

[84] Senator Brownback, May 22, 2003.

[85] Congressional Record, May 22, 2003: D576. See also, "Congress Votes to Keep the Abortion Ban on Bases," *Washington Post*, May 23, 2003: A7.

[86] Congressional Record, May 19, 2004: H3358.

[87] Congressional Record, June 22, 2004: S7152.

[88] Congressional Record, October 8, 2004: H9549.

[89] Congressional Record, May 25, 2005: H4009-H4013, H4017.

[90] Congressional Record, July 25, 2005, S8845.

[91] U.S. Congress, Senate, Armed Services Committee, National Defense Authorization Act for Fiscal Year 2011, S.Rept. 111-201, S. 3454, 111th Cong., 2nd Sess., June 4, 2010: 149.

[92] P.L. 112-81, SA 1120 was determined to be nongermane and SA 1121 was submitted on Nov. 17, 2011, with no further action listed in LIS.

INDEX

F

G

H

T

U

United States, v, 10, 11, 12, 26, 39, 45, 47,
  62, 71, 75, 77, 104, 125, 132, 133, 136,
  138, 143, 145, 146, 148, 149, 150, 151,
  153, 154, 155, 156, 158
updating, 98
upper respiratory infection, 69
urban, 119, 124
urban areas, 119
USA, 158
uterus, 107

V

VA health care beneficiaries, viii, 31, 33
vaccine, 110, 112, 127
variations, 98, 136, 154
Vatican, 154
veto, 139, 140, 146, 147, 150

victimization, 149
victims, 137, 156
Vietnam, viii, 32, 38, 42, 136
vision, 69
visual acuity, 106
vote, 132, 147, 148, 150, 152, 157

W

waiver, 90, 91, 114, 115, 116, 117, 118
war, 7, 34, 51, 71
Washington, 6, 42, 70, 71, 72, 115, 122,
  123, 124, 155, 156, 157, 158, 159
web, 13, 14, 15, 16, 28
wheezing, 69
wholesale, 111
Wisconsin, 5
worldwide, vii, 1, 5, 11, 141